WHAT DOCTORS DON'T TELL YOU

ARTHRITIS

WHAT DOCTORS DON'T TELL YOU

ARTHRITIS

Drug-Free
Alternatives to
Prevent and Reverse
Arthritis

Editor
Lynne McTaggart

HAY HOUSE

Carlsbad, California • New York City • London
Sydney •Johannesburg • Vancouver • New Delhi

First published and distributed in the United Kingdom by:
Hay House UK Ltd, Astley House, 33 Notting Hill Gate, London W11 3JQ
Tel: +44 (0)20 3675 2450; Fax: +44 (0)20 3675 2451; www.hayhouse.co.uk

Published and distributed in the United States of America by:
Hay House Inc., PO Box 5100, Carlsbad, CA 92018-5100
Tel: (1) 760 431 7695 or (800) 654 5126
Fax: (1) 760 431 6948 or (800) 650 5115; www.hayhouse.com

Published and distributed in Australia by:
Hay House Australia Ltd, 18/36 Ralph St, Alexandria NSW 2015
Tel: (61) 2 9669 4299; Fax: (61) 2 9669 4144; www.hayhouse.com.au

Published and distributed in the Republic of South Africa by:
Hay House SA (Pty) Ltd, PO Box 990, Witkoppen 2068
info@hayhouse.co.za; www.hayhouse.co.za

Published and distributed in India by:
Hay House Publishers India, Muskaan Complex, Plot No.3, B-2,
Vasant Kunj, New Delhi 110 070
Tel: (91) 11 4176 1620; Fax: (91) 11 4176 1630; www.hayhouse.co.in

Distributed in Canada by:
Raincoast Books, 2440 Viking Way, Richmond, B.C. V6V 1N2
Tel: (1) 604 448 7100; Fax: (1) 604 270 7161; www.raincoast.com

A catalogue record for this book is available from the British Library.

ISBN: 978-1-78180-338-7

Printed and bound by CPI Group (UK) Ltd, Croydon, CR0 4YY

For our readers

CONTENTS

Part III: Alternative Treatments for Arthritis

ABOUT WHAT DOCTORS DON'T TELL YOU

What Doctors Don't Tell You is one of the world's most respected information resources about safe and effective treatments in alternative medicine and the dangers and limitations of much of conventional medicine.

WDDTY, as it's popularly known, is a monthly glossy magazine, an award-winning website (www.wddty.com) and a community of people around the world seeking out safer and effective therapies.

Its hallmark is health information backed by exhaustive scientific research; in fact, readers have come to place such trust in the accuracy of WDDTY that information in its pages has even been cited in courts of law.

WDDTY's research has helped many thousands of people overcome a vast variety of conditions and regain their health, while many more have maintained their health, thanks to WDDTY's broad reach of research, which also encompasses nutrition, exercise and other lifestyle issues.

It was started in 1989 by its two editors, Lynne McTaggart, bestselling author of *The Field*, *The Intention Experiment* and *The Bond*, and her husband, Bryan Hubbard, a former *Financial Times* journalist and author of *The Untrue Story of You*.

McTaggart and Hubbard launched their publication in 1989 out of a sense of frustration with conventional medicine, and a desire to tell others about its shortcomings, after an odyssey of Lynne's to solve her own puzzling health problem. When nothing – from conventional or alternative medicine – seemed to help, she began doing her own research into what appeared to be the most appropriate therapy and sought out the doctor, a nutritional pioneer, most likely to help her. In the process, she realized that patients were more likely to get better if they were put in charge of their own decision-making.

Lynne's eyes had first been opened to the limitation of conventional medicine by one of America's leading doctors. Before creating What Doctors Don't Tell You, Lynne, as editor of a national newspaper syndicate, launched the national column of the legendary Dr Robert Mendelsohn, one of the first doctors to blow the whistle on medical practices.

WDDTY began life as an eight-page newsletter and has evolved into a glossy international magazine that has attracted many thousands of readers and subscribers. It is currently published in the UK and the USA, and under licence in 12 other countries.

Its editorial panel includes 12 noted pioneers of nutritional, environmental and alternative medicine, nine of whom are medical doctors.

The launch of WDDTY in the UK soon got the press's attention. *The Times* called it 'a voice in the silence,' while *The Observer* said it 'rang the alarm bells on procedures long before they became the stuff of national panic'.

WDDTY has also published 20 books on health conditions, and has several audio courses available.

The What Doctors Don't Tell You website has twice won Most Popular Health Website of the Year award, landing more votes than such well-known sites as BUPA and the National Health Service. It attracts hundreds of thousands of visitors every month, who use its searchable 10,000-page database for vital information about overcoming virtually every condition without drugs or surgery.

In 2015, WDDTY Publishing Ltd was awarded Ethical Business of the Year by popular reader vote, in a competition conducted by the magazine *Kindred Spirit*.

Over the years WDDTY has been acknowledged as one of the world's very best health resources by several commentators, including leading publisher and health campaigner Burton Goldberg, leading holistic healer Dr John Diamond, the Holistic Health Library and UK allergy specialist Dr John Mansfield.

To find out more and to subscribe to the magazine, visit www.wddty.com.

INTRODUCTION

Most of us accept that, as we get older, we'll be more likely to start suffering from aches and pains. Even in early middle age, many people suffer back pain that is so severe that they have to take time off work.

We may not even call it arthritis: it might start out as a twinge that just gets progressively worse. Only half of us even bother to see a doctor about our aches and pains, most likely because, like the medical profession, we are resigned to accept it as an unwelcome consequence of growing older. It's just 'wear and tear', as our family doctor might put it.

But these 'worn-out' joints have reached pandemic levels in the Western world. A chronic condition that bedevils conventional medicine, it's one of the most common diseases associated with old age, and one of the biggest causes of disability at any time of life.

An estimated 10 per cent of the world's population over the age of 60 currently displays osteoarthritis symptoms. Arthritis can strike at any age, within any ethnic population – although according to the Centers for Disease Control and Prevention in the USA, Hispanics, Asians and Pacific Islanders are almost half as likely to develop the disease as non-Hispanic whites and non-Hispanic Afro-Americans.

According to the National Health Interview Survey in 2011, more than 50 million people in the United States reported having been diagnosed with some form of arthritis, including some 300,000 children. The situation is no better in Britain, where unofficial estimates suggest that nine out of every 10 people will suffer from it in some form before they die.

Actually, arthritis isn't a proper disease but an umbrella term that describes a collection of symptoms with many potential causes. Arthritis simply means inflammation of one or more joints in the body. Pain and stiffness are the most universal symptoms of arthritis, and the pain, which can be severe, is as crippling as the physiological debilitation itself. Arthritic pain is caused by joint inflammation and, when the cartilage that protects joints breaks down, the rubbing action when unprotected bone meets bone. The word derives from the Greek: *arth* means 'joint' and *itis* means 'inflammation'.

This general term covers some 200 specific forms of the condition, ranging from osteoarthritis, which is the most prevalent, to rheumatoid arthritis, juvenile arthritis, ankylosing spondylitis, gout and systemic lupus erythematosus (SLE). Doctors even use this catch-all term now to describe musculoskeletal conditions such as polymyalgia rheumatica or any disease of the bones and joints, back pain, osteoporosis, and soft-tissue rheumatism.

Despite the common nature of the problem and the considerable amounts of money spent on researching it, medicine has found no real answers to arthritis in any of its widely varied forms.

Conventional treatment for arthritis conditions, unsurprisingly, focuses on the use of pharmaceutical medications to mitigate symptoms and hopefully to slow the progress of the disease.

The typical arthritis patient is likely to be offered a giant arsenal of drugs falling into three broad treatment categories: painkillers, anti-inflammatories and 'disease modifiers'. The latter are drugs that claim to halt or even reverse the arthritis process – a term and outlook that seem far too optimistic, considering the consensus view that current drugs on offer fail to control disease adequately in many patients.[1]

In fact, drug side effects accompany most standard treatments, many of them as debilitating as the disease they purport to treat, and not infrequently life-threatening, particularly as some patients end up being prescribed a variety of drugs for upwards of 30 years or more.

Surgery, of course, is the 'last stop' treatment when all else fails – and the conventional 'all else' often does fail. Approximately 500,000 knee replacements and more than 175,000 hip replacements are performed annually, in America alone, and those numbers are on the rise. According to a study presented at the American Academy of Orthopaedic Surgeons in 2006, the number of hip replacements was anticipated to increase by 174 per cent and knee replacements by 673 per cent over the next 20 years.

This book will be something of a revelation if you're an arthritis sufferer who's been told that nothing can be done for you other than to take a painkiller and wait until you're a candidate for joint replacement surgery. You don't have to suffer in silence as the arthritis gets progressively worse. As you'll discover in these pages, there's a large array of options open to you – including dietary changes, alternative and complementary medicine, supplements, body and mind therapies – many with a proven track record of success.

Our findings should give you great hope. There are many things you can do to overcome or lessen your symptoms, and some of these may even reverse the disease itself. These ideas are not based on the case studies of a handful of people, but are the result of painstaking scientific research, used successfully on thousands of sufferers like yourself.

Being healthy, staying healthy and getting healthy require information, effort and frequently a willingness to go against conventional thinking in healthcare. In too many instances the conventional approach is simply a process of symptom management, created by an industry that stands to gain primarily from lifelong drug management, not from cures.

This book will give you the necessary information to make informed choices for your health and well-being with regard to arthritis – how to prevent it and what to do to get on the path to healing if you're already dealing with it.

In the following pages, may you begin your journey to better health.

/IIIIIIIIIIIIIIIIIIIIIIIIIIIIIIIIIIIIIIIIIIIIII

Part I

THE CONVENTIONAL APPROACH

Chapter 1

MODERN MEDICINE'S THEORY OF ARTHRITIS

A rthritis isn't a new disease. It has plagued humankind ever since we've been able to keep any sort of records; in fact, some of the mummies of ancient Egypt showed signs of it. And, unlike so many chronic conditions, it isn't confined to the West: most nations of the world are recording increasing levels of the disease.

One phenomenon of modern times is the extraordinary increase in the incidence of arthritis. It's been estimated that nine out of 10 of us will suffer from some form of it to a lesser or greater extent before we die. So why has it become so prevalent in recent years? And have the 10 per cent of people who *don't* develop the condition anything to teach us?

In the early part of the 20th century, scientists were convinced that arthritis was a chronic infection of the joints. This has given way to more recent theories, particularly the idea that arthritis is largely hereditary – a genetic tendency – or else an infection, caused by the bacterial micro-organism *Mycoplasma*, or even a malfunction of the body's metabolic and immune systems. All agree, though, that the exact cause can't yet be identified with any certainty.

Statistics do show that autoimmune diseases such as rheumatoid arthritis and Crohn's disease often run in families. However, of the three theories, the notion that arthritis is a malfunctioning immune system is the most favoured and the most actively researched in laboratories; this is a credible possibility for autoimmune conditions like rheumatoid arthritis, but an inadequate explanation for all of the diseases lumped under the arthritis umbrella (*see below*).

Types of arthritis

The catch-all term arthritis can be broken down into six specific disease groups:

⇨　Non-articular rheumatism
　　　– Soft-tissue rheumatism
　　　– Back pain and disc lesions
　　　– Shoulder, hand and foot problems

⇨　Degenerative
　　　– Osteoarthritis

⇨　Inflammatory
　　　– Rheumatoid arthritis
　　　– Polyarthritis
　　　– Childhood polyarthritis
　　　– Ankylosing spondylitis
　　　– Psoriatic arthritis

⇨   Connective tissue disease
- Polymyalgia rheumatica
- Systemic lupus erythematosus
- Schleroderma

⇨   Crystal arthritis
- Gout and pseudogout

⇨   Bone disorders
- Osteoporosis
- Rickets and ostemalacia
- Paget's disease

Since arthritis is a misleading, catch-all term for a variety of diseases of the bones, joints and tissues, it's not surprising that there is also a range of different causes. However, before looking at some of the specific arthritic diseases, it's important first to understand what constitutes a healthy joint.

Joints comprise bone with a layer of smooth, less brittle cartilage known as the articular cartilage, which is separated from the opposite bone and cartilage by a lubricating synovial fluid, contained within a synovial membrane (synovium).

The bone consists of a matrix of collagen, a form of protein, which binds together calcium, the main constituent of bone and phosphorus. The cartilage protects the bone ends, and is composed of proteoglycans, a type of mucopolysaccharide made from protein and carbohydrate.

Types of arthritis

Under the catch-all term 'arthritis' the following conditions are included:

Osteoarthritis

Osteoarthritis is the most common form of the disease, affecting more than 70 per cent of adults between the ages of 55 and 78, the majority being women. Doctors mainly view osteoarthritis as a 'normal' degenerative process related to age, or a condition that commonly strikes after infection or injury, or among people who are overweight.

Osteoarthritis, also known as 'wear-and-tear' arthritis, affects the cartilage of joints, causing it to break down. The job of this tough, elastic tissue is to cover the bones that adjoin at every joint, reducing their friction as they rub together. As the cartilage breaks down, it becomes frayed and rough, and the protective space between the bones decreases. During movement, the bones of the joint rub against each other, causing pain. Over time the cartilage dries out, becoming cracked and pitted, no longer allowing smooth movement of the joint. When cartilage wears away in a weight-bearing joint such as the hip or knee, this can produce severe pain, deformity and loss of mobility.

The disease is most commonly found in the hands, but it also affects weight-bearing joints such as the knees and hips, and also the joints of the spine.

In the early stages, you just feel stiffness, and movement may become a little difficult. Patients may not suffer any pain at this point. However, in the late stages of the condition, bone spurs called osteophytes – abnormal bone projections that develop along the edges of bones – can form. The cartilage can even disappear completely in severe cases, leaving the bone ends exposed. A common feature of osteoarthritis is hard knobs called Heberden's nodes, which develop around the edges of the finger joints, caused by the breakdown of cartilage.

This variety of arthritis can be detected from blood tests, such as the erythrocyte sedimentation rate (ESR), which measures the speed at which red blood cells settle in a tube, indicating the amount of inflammation.

X-rays are used to reveal the degree of deterioration in the joints – and doctors tend to look out for joint narrowing and the presence of bone spurs, although these can only help to determine how much bone and cartilage damage has already been done.

Rheumatoid arthritis

Rheumatoid arthritis (RA) is also a chronic inflammatory disease, typically affecting the synovial lining of joints, most often in the hands and feet, but also in multiple joints throughout the body, especially elbows, wrists, ankles and knees. It also attacks shoulders and hip joints. Unlike osteoarthritis, where the joint itself breaks down, RA causes the synovium, or membrane lining around the joints, to become inflamed, which attracts more joint fluid to ease it. Eventually the joint becomes swollen, stiff and warm because of the increased blood flow.

Classified as an autoimmune disease, RA occurs when white blood cells produce antibodies that attack and destroy healthy tissue instead of attacking infection and disease. Doctors have no idea why this happens, but the chronic release of antibodies over time thickens the synovium and damages the cartilage and bone of the affected joints, causing crippling pain, deformity and eventual bone erosion. Other symptoms can include tiredness and muscle pain.

RA strikes roughly three times as many women as men and can affect any age group, although those younger than 35 years are a very low-risk group. Signs and symptoms of rheumatoid arthritis may include:

⇨ Sore, swollen joints that feel very warm to the touch

⇨ Morning stiffness

⇨ Rheumatoid nodules – firm bumps of tissue on the arms

⇨ Low-grade fever, fatigue and weight loss

An average of one in 10 patients are thought to recover within two years. However, RA is known to 'come and go' frequently, with varying periods of acute symptoms followed by apparent remission.

Gout

Also known as crystal arthritis, gout is one of the most common types of inflammatory arthritis, affecting 1.4 per cent of adults in the UK, or an estimated 225,000 men and 57,000 women. An acute form of inflammatory arthritis usually affecting the metatarsal-phalangeal joint at the base of the big toe, gout causes intense pain in the affected joints, which can also include wrist and finger joints.

Gout is a disease of middle age, affecting 15 times more men than women, and has long been linked to overindulgence of rich foods and alcohol consumption, although alternative practitioners have found that food allergies and the use of diuretic drugs, often prescribed for heart conditions, can also trigger the disorder.

Pain and swelling occur when minute crystals form in the joint space. The crystals are caused by excess uric acid in the body. The immune system attacks these crystals with phagocytes (scavenger cells,) and the toxic by-product of this clash causes the joint inflammation. Patients receive their first warning signal when they experience an arthritic attack in one of their big toes or one of the other common sites, when the joint becomes tender and painful. Classic signs are redness, swelling and attacks of severe pain.

Ankylosing spondylitis

Spondylitis, meaning 'inflammation of the joints of the spine,' affects the point where ligaments and tendons join the bone. This is the most common type of arthritis to affect young and middle-aged men, occurring most often between the sacrum (the last bone in the spine) and the pelvis. The classic sufferer has a rigid, painful spine and difficulty holding up the head when walking. Along with severe back pain, another warning sign of the disease is the development of iritis, an inflammation of the iris of the eye.

Systemic lupus erythematosus (SLE)

This disease, which usually strikes young women, can affect any joint. It's thought to be genetic or caused by drugs and even to have some relation to sunlight, although it is generally accepted that SLE is an autoimmune condition. A red rash over the nose and cheeks is a warning sign.

Polymyalgia rheumatica

Polymyalgia rheumatica is mostly a muscle disorder, but can affect the joints of people over 50 years old. It attacks the hips and shoulders and causes tenderness and distinct muscle pain.

Psoriatic arthritis

Doctors have found a strong link between arthritis and the skin disorder psoriasis. Psoriatic arthritis occurs in 7 per cent of patients with psoriasis, and 20 per cent of patients with psoriatic arthritis have psoriasis. At times, the only symptom is a change in the nails – either pitting or discoloration. The condition usually affects only one or two joints.

Infectious or micro-organism-related arthritis

This form of arthritis comes from a bacterial, viral or fungal infection that spreads from another part of the body. The types found include viral arthritis (caused by a virus such as rubella), septic arthritis (due to bacteria such as staphylococci) and rheumatic fever (from a throat infection caused by streptococci or the like). However, medical scientists are also just beginning to make the link between joint pain and persistent unwanted guests such as parasites (*see Chapter 6*).

Symptoms of infectious arthritis include intense pain in the joints, and redness and swelling there, along with chills and fever.

Post-traumatic arthritis

Post-traumatic arthritis is a form of osteoarthritis that develops after an injury, such as a wrist fracture or dislocation of the shoulder.

The conventional view of causes

Osteoarthritis, the mildest and most common form of the disease, is blamed by medicine on 'wear and tear,' and wrongly viewed as an inevitable consequence of old age. However, when it comes to rheumatoid arthritis and the many other forms of the disease, medicine admits it's at a loss to understand the causes.

Very early studies have drawn a link between, on the one hand, vitamin D deficiencies associated with lack of sunshine and, on the other, the by-product of other autoimmune diseases such as Crohn's disease and multiple sclerosis (MS) as RA is generally considered an autoimmune disease. A study profiling 461 women with rheumatoid arthritis comparing them to 9,220 healthy controls revealed that women in the northeastern states of America, such as Vermont, New Hampshire and southern Maine, which have less sunshine than more southerly states, are more likely to suffer from rheumatoid arthritis.[1] But so far no definite conclusions have been formed.

Evidence is accumulating for a link between rubella immunization and the development of arthralgia, or general joint stiffness, or arthritis. In a recent randomized, placebo-controlled trial, 30 per cent of women given the rubella vaccine developed acute, short-term joint problems, compared with 20 per cent of those given a placebo. The groups were followed up at one, three, six, nine and 12 months after immunizations. Although the gap between the two groups in terms of severity of symptoms did narrow over time, the authors still conclude that some women are more susceptible and may experience arthritic symptoms after rubella immunization.[2]

The truth is that there's no consensus within the medical community on the causes of *any* of the forms of arthritis, which is why its only response is to prescribe painkillers and anti-inflammatory drugs to control the symptoms.

:::

Chapter 2

FIRST-LINE PAIN TREATMENT

It's a scene that's played out every day in doctors' surgeries. You've been suffering from a nagging pain in your knee for some days, and the stiffness just won't go away. At your first visit, the doctor arranged for you to visit your local hospital for X-rays and a simple blood test. Now the results are back.

'You've got early-stage osteoarthritis,' says your doctor. 'I'm afraid it's all part of growing older, just the wear and tear of life.'

He might suggest some exercise before reaching for his pad to write out a prescription. This is the only response that medicine has to arthritis: a drug, usually an NSAID (non-steroidal anti-inflammatory drug) to alleviate pain.

The drugs used to control the symptoms are known as 'first-line' drugs, and include NSAIDs, which are claimed to reduce swelling in the joints, and the simple painkillers known as analgesics.

Conventional first-line medication

The most common and popular over-the-counter (OTC) analgesic (pain relief) medication for chronic pain is the old standby, aspirin (acetylsalicylic acid). The oldest and most popular analgesic on the market, aspirin is a classic NSAID (non-steroidal anti-inflammatory drug).

Paracetamol, sold as Calpol or Panadol in the UK (acetaminophen in the USA, sold as Tylenol and Excedrin), came onto the market in 1955. Although often used for arthritis pain, it's assumed to have slightly less effect on pain from inflammation than aspirin and other, newer NSAIDs such as ibuprofen (with tradenames like Anadin, Arthrofen, Nurofen, Brufen, Calprofen, Galprofen, Ibuleve, Motrin, Orbifen and Advil). And, in fact, a study of 184 patients found that large (2,400mg) and small (1,200mg) daily doses of the NSAID ibuprofen worked about the same as high daily doses (4,000mg) of paracetamol in controlling pain and inflammation.[1]

Aspirin, ibuprofen and all the ibuprofen 'clones' are non-selective NSAIDs that supposedly work by inhibiting two enzymes that are involved with inflammation: cyclooxygenase-1 and cyclooxygenase-2 (COX-1 and COX-2). The body produces COX enzymes wherever they are needed (in almost every organ of the body) to control the production of chemicals called prostaglandins, which, among other things, reduce pain by interrupting or suppressing pain signals carried along the nerves. Unfortunately, prostaglandins carry out a number of other complex functions in the body as well, and interfering with them causes a number of different side effects, including indigestion and stomach ulcers.

As the 'anti-inflammatory' element in their generic name suggests, these are painkillers that are also supposed to reduce swelling. However, as osteoarthritis doesn't always involve swelling around the joints, it could be argued that, of the 24 million prescriptions for NSAIDs handed out in Britain alone, most could be replaced by a simple painkiller. Furthermore, there's a question mark over their efficacy as anti-inflammatories: Dr Peter Gøtzsche, head of the Cochrane Collaboration in Denmark, who was a researcher on the early NSAID drug trials, admitted that some of the initial studies on NSAIDs were manipulated because they showed no benefit in reducing inflammation over simple painkillers.[2]

While NSAIDs have undoubtedly brought pain relief to some arthritis sufferers, they may also be accelerating the condition, especially in the case of osteoarthritis. Studies have shown that NSAIDs speed the progress of the disease, largely because they inhibit cartilage repair and promote cartilage destruction.[3]

NANS: the 'non-anti-inflammatories'

If you're less than happy with the drugs you take for osteoarthritis, Dr Peter Gøtzsche, head of the Scandinavian arm of the Cochrane Collaboration and one of its founders, believes he knows why. He's made the extraordinary charge that non-steroidal anti-inflammatory drugs (NSAIDs) don't, in fact, reduce inflammation.

In his book *Deadly Medicines and Organised Crime: How Big Pharma has Corrupted Healthcare*, he states: 'The idea of an anti-inflammatory effect of NSAIDs is a hoax, like so many other myths about drugs that the drug companies have invented and marketed.'[4]

Gøtzsche has conducted extensive studies into non-steroidal anti-inflammatories, beginning from the time he was medical director at Astra-Syntex in 1977. Astra had produced naproxen, an early NSAID. When Gøtzsche investigated the actions of various NSAIDs, he discovered that drug companies were manipulating information about this entire class of drugs, giving doctors the impression, through inference and with no supporting data, that NSAIDs were better than paracetamol (acetaminophen) because they didn't just reduce pain, but also reduced inflammation.

When Gøtzsche and a group of orthopaedic surgeons carried out their own independent study of naproxen, they found that the drug had no effect on reducing inflammation in patients with twisted ankles: patients recovered faster simply by keeping the affected limb moving.

After studying some 244 NSAIDs in trials, Gøtzsche uncovered an overwhelming amount of bias favouring any given sponsoring company's drug over the control drug.[5] Then, in his own studies, the drugs failed to work as anti-inflammatories: compared with placebos, they had no effect on swollen finger joints in patients with rheumatoid arthritis.

But the most scandalous aspect of the NSAID trials, according to Gøtzsche, was that certain dangers associated with the drugs, many of which cause gastrointestinal bleeding and heart attacks, were minimized.

Furthermore, he discovered that doubling the dose, as patients have often been encouraged to do with all NSAIDs, produced negligible benefits, yet twice the amount of harm, including an increased risk of bleeding ulcers and even death.[6]

Death by aspirin

For all their commonness and assumed benevolence, aspirin and other common non-selective NSAIDs may be major killers – ones that few of us ever suspect.

For decades aspirin has been promoted as a relatively benign drug. The American Association of Poison Control Centers receives reports of just 59 aspirin deaths in the USA each year, while researchers put the rate for all painkilling NSAIDs at around 7,600 deaths a year.[7] Either way, doctors have argued that these figures represent an acceptable risk in relation to the benefits – including the many additional thousands who might otherwise have died from heart disease if not for taking these magic white pills.

But scientists are now discovering that we've been shockingly misled by the medical community. Far from being benign, aspirin, ibuprofen and other NSAIDs cause serious – and, in some cases, fatal – gastrointestinal (GI) bleeding. According to C.J. Hawkey, a researcher at Queen's Medical Centre, University Hospital in Nottingham, 'NSAIDs account for more reports of drug-related toxicity than any other class of drugs.'[8] Their most widespread adverse effects are on the gastrointestinal tract, where they are responsible for more than a staggering 50 per cent of all cases of ulcer bleeding and perforation, says Hawkey – cases so severe that the arthritis patient may be hospitalized or even die. It's been estimated that NSAID side effects on the gut cause more than 16,000 deaths per year in the USA alone.[9]

And researchers have discovered another worrying side effect of aspirin, ibuprofen and other NSAIDs: they may be a major cause of stroke among the elderly. However, it isn't just the elderly who are affected. Recent studies show that ibuprofen and similar NSAIDs could treble the risk of strokes and double the chance of heart attack in those taking heavy doses over the long term in the general population.[10]

The true casualty rate

The US Food and Drug Administration's own best estimate is that 200,000 cases of gastric bleeding occur with NSAIDs each year, including 10,000–20,000 deaths. In the UK, some 4,000 people die each year from these drugs – twice the number of deaths from asthma. Besides ulcers, even the 'safest' of NSAIDs, ibuprofen, can cause colitis. The NSAIDS indomethacin, naproxen and a sustained-release preparation of ketoprofen all can cause perforations of the colon.

Most of these deaths are slipping under the radar and not being associated with NSAIDs at all. Researchers at the Eastern Virginia Medical School were among the first to make an alarming discovery when they interviewed patients at a clinic that specializes in GI problems. Nearly one in five patients were taking aspirin or some other painkilling NSAID, but not reporting the fact to the medical staff because it wasn't regarded as significant.[11]

'This reflects a common misperception,' said Dr David Johnson, one of the researchers, 'that these medications are insignificant or benign when actually their chronic use, particularly among the elderly and those with conditions such as arthritis, is linked to serious and potentially fatal GI injury and bleeding.'

If the researchers' estimates are correct, the worldwide NSAID death toll could be as high as 100,000 individuals every year – with another 500,000 needing hospital care to treat a serious reaction to the drugs.[12]

Equally worrying is the effect of this class of drugs on people over 75 years of age. Far from protecting them against stroke, it appears these NSAIDs are causing just such an attack, often with fatal or disabling results. Researchers at Oxford University have discovered that NSAIDs have caused a sevenfold increase in intracerebral haemorrhagic stroke – bleeding within the brain – during the past 25 years among groups of elderly patients who participated in their trial.[13]

Research team leader Professor Peter Rothwell says that NSAIDs may soon replace high blood pressure as the leading cause of intracerebral haemorrhagic stroke, especially among those aged over 75. 'There are elderly people who take aspirin as a lifestyle choice and, in that situation, the trials have shown there's no benefit. And what our study suggests is that, particularly in the very elderly, the risks of aspirin outweigh the benefits.'

In Rothwell's study, researchers assessed the records of stroke victims between 1981 and 1985, and again between 2002 and 2006. While the overall rate of stroke caused by high blood pressure had dropped by 65 per cent between those two periods, the rate among the over-75s remained the same, mainly because there'd been an increase in the number of strokes among patients taking blood-thinners such as aspirin.

The team discovered that the use of these drugs had increased dramatically, especially among healthy people who were taking them as a preventative.[14] Between 1981 and 1985, only 4 per cent of patients were taking a blood-thinner, a figure that rose to 40 per cent in the more recent time period.

Ignoring the warning signs

Apparently, the true dangers of aspirin have been known for some time: it's just that no one in the medical community has been prepared to do anything about it. Scientists from the West Midlands Regional Health Authority in Birmingham were among the first to raise the warning flag in the mid-1990s when they investigated the reasons why people were in hospital for treatment of bleeding peptic ulcer.

At that time, they discovered that 12.8 per cent of the 1,121 patients being investigated were 'regular' users of aspirin, which they defined as five days a week for at least a month. When they compared these patients against other patients with the same problem, but who were not regularly taking aspirin, it was evident that taking the NSAID had increased the risk of hospitalization for bleeding peptic ulcer by 2.3 times at a low dose of just 75mg, and by up to 3.9 times at the more standard dose of 300mg.[15] The 300mg dose is the recommended level for 'just in case' prophylactic use against heart disease.

Not only can the use of NSAIDs lead to gastrointestinal problems, it can also cause blurred or diminished vision, Parkinson's disease, and hair and fingernail loss. These drugs can also damage the liver and kidneys, and increase the risk of high blood pressure (hypertension), especially when taken in large doses. Instead of issuing warnings, one drug industry response to these side effects was to create topical NSAID lotions, which are supposed to take away the pain of arthritis while avoiding the drawbacks of their oral cousins.

However, when a group of scientists at Nottingham University studied the topical lotions in depth, they found they don't really work. The group analysed 13 trials comparing topical NSAIDs with placebo treatments and NSAIDs given orally as tablets. Although the topical creams offered better pain relief at first, after two weeks they offered no more relief than the fake (placebo) treatments. They also caused a number of side effects of their own, such as itching, rash and burning. The researchers concluded that 'No evidence supports the long-term use of topical NSAIDs in osteoarthritis.'[16]

Who is most at risk?

The research indicates that approximately twice as many men as women end up in hospital with aspirin/NSAID-related gastric problems. And individuals who take several NSAIDs in combination increase their risk of having a serious GI reaction. In a separate study, researchers who examined patients' records from databases in the UK and Spain found that 60 per cent of those who suffered a GI reaction from an NSAID were aged over 60. Thirteen per cent were using several NSAIDs in combination. Also worth noting is that 6 per cent had a recent history of peptic ulcers – even though patients with pre-existing GI problems are not supposed to be taking an NSAID in the first place.[17]

But perhaps the group of people most at risk are those taking the lethal drug combination of an NSAID with a SSRI (selective serotonin reuptake inhibitor) type of antidepressant such as Prozac, Zoloft or Paxil – a common drug cocktail among arthritis sufferers who are often prescribed an NSAID to ease joint pain and inflammation and an SSRI to ease their mild depression.

Researchers from the University of East Anglia made this discovery when they carried out a meta-analysis of four trials involving a total of 153,000 patients who were taking either an SSRI or an NSAID, or a combination of the two. Patients who took just the SSRI increased the risk of a GI reaction 2.4 times, and those taking just an NSAID had a 3.2 times greater risk.[18] However, when the two drugs were combined, the risk of upper GI haemorrhage increased by 6.3 times. This means that potentially a patient only has to take the combination around 82 times before suffering a serious gastrointestinal reaction – in other words, less than three months into treatment if the combination of the two drugs is taken on a daily basis, which it usually is.

'Before I did this study, I didn't worry at all when I saw patients who were on combinations of SSRIs and NSAIDs,' said lead researcher Dr Yoon K. Loke. 'Now that I have seen the fairly substantial excess risk, physicians should review the patients' charts – do they need to be on these drugs at all, or are there safer alternatives?'

Gastrointestinal problems linked with NSAIDs have been known for a long time – even if the severity and extent have only recently been revealed – and manufacturers have tried to reduce the risk by producing versions that are either enteric-coated – given a polymer coating to keep the pill intact in the stomach, allowing for easier absorption by the small intestine – or buffered, which coats the standard pill with a substance that neutralizes stomach acid.

But far from reducing the GI risk, these coatings appear actually to increase it. Researchers from the Boston University School of Medicine interviewed 550 hospital patients with major upper gastrointestinal bleeding about their aspirin use. To their surprise, they found that those who'd regularly taken buffered aspirin were at far greater risk of developing GI problems than were those taking regular aspirin tablets. At doses greater than 325mg, patients taking the buffered tablets were seven times more likely to develop GI problems compared with a fivefold increased risk among those taking the standard pills.[19]

The story of aspirin

Aspirin holds an unusual place in trademark law. As 'Aspirin' with a capital 'A', it's a protected brand, owned by Bayer, the German pharmaceutical giant.

Aspirin's principal ingredient is salicylic acid, derived from the bark of the willow tree (recognized by Hippocrates as a pain-reliever and antipyretic, or fever-reducer, as long ago as the 5th century BC) and from the herb meadowsweet. Chemists at Bayer successfully synthesized salicylic acid with the common chemical acetic anhydride, giving Aspirin its generic name. As 'aspirin', it's a generic drug that can be used in countries where Aspirin is not trademark-protected. Around 50 other over-the-counter preparations contain aspirin, labelled as 'Aspirin' or ASA, Aspirin's 'official' generic name, acetylsalicylic acid.

Bayer began marketing this drug in 1899, along with another of the company's therapeutic discoveries: heroin. Despite its widespread use and popularity, no one understood how aspirin worked until 1971, when the British pharmacologist John Vane found that it suppresses the production of prostaglandins and thromboxanes, hormones that regulate many physiological functions, including the transmission of pain signals to the brain.

Current global consumption is 35,000 tons of aspirin every year – amounting to around 100 billion tablets – a figure that's increasing annually by 15 per cent.

Not for children

Aspirin is no longer recommended for children under the age of 12 because of the very real danger of children taking aspirin developing Reye's syndrome, a rare, often fatal disorder primarily seen in children recovering from a viral illness but also linked with aspirin use.[20]

Despite this setback, ever since NSAIDs were given over-the-counter status in the 1990s, drug companies have pursued the lucrative kiddy market for painkillers. Currently ibuprofen has replaced paracetamol as the first port of call for treating juvenile pain. However, recent lawsuits in the USA on behalf of children who developed the rare and potentially fatal skin condition Stevens-Johnson syndrome (SJS) after taking children's ibuprofen could send ibuprofen into the same market tailspin as kiddy aspirin.

The cases include a nine-year-old California girl who died 20 months after taking children's Motrin, a seven-year-old who went blind two months after taking the same drug and a three-year-old who died a week after taking just a few doses of kiddy Advil.

SJS causes painful blistering of the skin. The biggest concern is that it will progress to the more serious form of the illness, toxic epidermal necrolysis, or TEN, where the outermost layer of skin peels off. TEN is fatal in about a third of cases. The syndrome can also cause blisters, and even erosion and perforation of the cornea of the eye. Most cases of SJS are drug reactions: it should be added that virtually any drug can cause SJS.

Cases of SJS from NSAIDs are not confined to children. Currently, though, the US Food and Drug Administration is not requiring drug-makers – including those manufacturing NSAIDs – to put a warning on their products, largely because SJS is so rare. Stevens-Johnson syndrome supposedly affects one to six people per million in the USA. The official position is that labels should only mention the more common side effects such as gastrointestinal bleeding. At the moment, the FDA does not even require cases of SJS to be reported.

The FDA claims it has received, thus far, some 150 reports of SJS in patients who'd taken ibuprofen. The Stevens-Johnson Syndrome Foundation in Westminster, Colorado, has warned parents to stop giving their children ibuprofen or any other drugs if they develop a rash (an early sign of SJS) or blisters on the ears, nose and genitals, or develop sores inside their mouth.

Other potential side effects from ibuprofen include heartburn, abdominal pain, nausea, ulcers and gastrointestinal bleeding, increased problems in patients with ulcers, mental depression, ringing in the ears (tinnitus), weight gain, swelling in the lower extremities, vomiting, changes in eyesight or hearing, nosebleeds, drowsiness, confusion and constipation.

Why NSAIDs cause side effects

Besides all the gut problems, researchers at the Johns Hopkins University School of Medicine say that common NSAID painkillers can cause a wide range of other unsuspected problems because, as new research has found, the drugs attack enzymes within cell membranes and cause unpredictable side effects in different parts of the body.

Researchers tested the effects of three prescription NSAIDs – flurbiprofen, indomethacin and sulindac – on human cells. The effect was greatest if the drug was administered for lengthy periods or in large doses. Over-the-counter painkillers didn't have the same damaging effects on enzymes.[21]

Cox-2 inhibitors

In the heady world of the pharmaceutical industry, the most profitable industry in the world, the pressure is always intense to develop new products that will revolutionize treatment in a particular area and redefine the marketplace.

No area offers more potential for major commercial success than something that will take away the pain of arthritis. Pharmaceutical corporations have been so desperate to find a breakthrough for arthritis pain that they've even experimented with a chemotherapy cocktail originally developed to combat non-Hodgkin's lymphoma – a drug so toxic it can cause acute respiratory failure within an hour of taking it.[22]

Enter the COX-2 inhibitors, the fair-haired boys of arthritis treatment, the 'super-aspirin' drugs that were marketed as the ultimate pain-reliever with no side effects attached. Indeed, the first two to be launched, celecoxib (Celebrex) and rofecoxib (Vioxx) (virtually all of these drugs have an 'x' in their names), became the most successful drugs in medical history almost overnight, snatching the mantle from Viagra.

COX-2 selective inhibitors primarily block the COX-2 enzyme. Selective non-steroidal anti-inflammatory drugs like these were designed to improve upon the usual NSAIDs, because of the latter's gastrointestinal (GI) side effects such as dyspepsia, peptic (oesophagus, stomach or duodenum) and intestinal ulcers, and a sometimes fatal haemorrhage.[23]

COX-2s were so popular in the arthritis market that doctors worldwide wrote more than 100 million prescriptions for Celebrex and Vioxx in the year 2000 alone. Vioxx had sales of $2.5 billion in 2003 and at one point an estimated 80 million people worldwide were taking the drug before it was pulled off the market by Merck in 2004 after disclosures that the company had withheld information from doctors and the public about the almost doubled risk of heart attack and stroke associated with high-dosage long-term use of the drug.

Celebrex, the only COX-2 selective NSAID drug still marketed in the UK and the USA, raked in more than $4 billion for Pfizer in the first six years of its launch.[24]

COX-2s and GI damage

Not only have the COX-2 drugs had a nasty track record for heart attack and stroke, most haven't even lived up to their original promise of providing a clean gastrointestinal bill of health for users. Researchers at Nottingham University have revealed that the COX-2s are just as bad as the original NSAIDs they were meant to replace. In a study of more than 9,400 patients diagnosed with a stomach ulcer or GI bleeding, the researchers found an increased risk of GI problems that was associated not only with the conventional NSAIDs but with the COX-2s as well.[25]

The safety risk was deemed slightly less for celecoxib (Celebrex), the only COX-2 selective NSAID left on the market after valdecoxib (Bextra), like rofecoxib (Vioxx), was recalled owing to concerns over cardiovascular problems. However, one study found that the patients taking celecoxib developed even more dyspepsia than those taking the conventional NSAID naproxen.[26]

One study, known as CLASS (Celecoxib Long-Term Arthritis Safety Study), claimed that it caused fewer GI side effects compared with the traditional NSAIDs. However, among patients taking aspirin as a just-in-case medicine to prevent heart disease, those given celecoxib as well had similar GI problems (such as ulcers) as those given diclofenac or ibuprofen.[27]

Numerous trials show that many of these drugs can cause ulcers.[28] And a Norwegian study concluded that COX-2s were actually more dangerous than NSAIDs and caused more side effects.[29] Valdecoxib (Bextra) was quickly linked to many life-threatening skin conditions, as well as potentially fatal anaphylactic (allergic) shock.

Drugs such as Celebrex have been linked to deaths from gastrointestinal ulcers and to heart problems. The Adenoma Prevention with Celecoxib (APC) study, co-sponsored by the US National Cancer Institute and Pfizer, which makes the drug, revealed that patients taking 200 mg of Celebrex twice daily were nearly two and a half times more likely to suffer a heart attack or stroke. This risk rose to 3.4 times with 400mg twice daily. Needless to say, the authors recommended that the study be discontinued before it ran its intended course.[30]

In terms of thromboembolic events (blood clots leading to stroke), Celebrex was no better than its banned sister Vioxx.[31]

As if all this weren't enough, taking COX-2 inhibitors has also been linked with kidney problems – frequently reported as footnotes to studies. According to one report, celecoxib resulted in hypertension, peripheral oedema and kidney failure in a quarter of all patients receiving the COX-2 drug.[32]

This should come as no surprise, because sodium excretion by the kidneys is at least partially assisted by COX-2 enzymes, and thus the use of COX-2 inhibitors can slow the elimination of sodium from the body. According to another study comparing the effects of rofecoxib with the conventional NSAID indomethacin during regular long-term use, both drugs hampered the kidney's ability to filter waste.

Consequently, patients on sodium-restricted diets and diuretic therapy, and individuals suffering from impaired kidney function, hypertension, congestive heart failure or liver disease, should avoid NSAID therapy, including COX-2 inhibitors.

Given the evidence linking COX-2s with an increased incidence of heart attack and stroke, some reconsideration of the cardiovascular safety profile of all NSAIDs – whether selective or non-selective – seems warranted. The FDA recommended back in 2005 that all such drugs carry a 'black box' warning for GI and cardiovascular risks,[33] and finally, in July 2015, it has strengthened those warnings in the light of evidence that not only can these drugs 'increase the chance of a heart attack or stroke, either of which can lead to death', but they aggravate the danger even in people 'without an underlying risk for cardiovascular disease'.[34]

||||||||||||||||||||||||||||||||||||||||||||

Chapter 3

SECOND-LINE TREATMENTS

U nlike first-line drugs, which are prescribed mainly to reduce pain and inflammation, second-line drugs are given in an attempt to modify the condition or to stop arthritis from progressing. Mainly prescribed for rheumatoid arthritis, this category is variously referred to as either DMARDs (disease-modifying antirheumatic drugs) or SAARDs (slow-acting antirheumatic drugs). Both refer to the same broad-brush group that includes: antimalarials and gold injections; synthetic agents such as methotrexate and sulphasalazine; anti-tumour necrosis factor agents (TNF blockers), such as etanercept and infliximab, which suppress the body's response to tumour necrosis factor, part of the inflammatory response; even powerful cytotoxic (cell-killing) immunosuppressant drugs, such as drugs developed for chemotherapy. Although not classified as 'disease-modifying', even corticosteroids (usually just referred to as steroids) – which regulate immune response and inflammation – get thrown at rheumatoid arthritis and polymyalgia rheumatica.

Unsurprisingly, these drugs too have had their problems, particularly with patients at risk of infection, and there have been reports of 'rare neurological and haematological events' (side effects related to the brain, nerves or blood).[1]

The use of all these types of drugs is based on the theory that arthritis is a malfunction of the immune system. Accordingly, doctors look to drugs that block basic immune-system processes to attempt to thwart or at least arrest the condition.

Second-line treatments, such as gold, methotrexate and sulphasalazine, are traditionally prescribed to rheumatoid arthritis sufferers once the disease is advanced. It is thought – or at least hoped – that these drugs can stop whatever autoimmune destruction is going on. Every case, however, is a decidedly hit-and-miss affair, with doctors coming upon something that seems to work in the course of treating something else. This treatment may slow down the progress of the disease, but also brings with it a host of side effects, including ulcers and life-threatening gastrointestinal problems. Many of the drugs the medical profession throws at sufferers are powerful immunosuppressants and cell-blockers developed to treat more serious and life-threatening conditions such as cancer.

Because first-line treatments like NSAIDs can only ease the pain, many specialists are now pushing SAARDs to the front, using them to slow the progress of rheumatoid arthritis and help to prevent damage to the joints.

Favourite among the SAARDs has always been gold, given either as an injection or in tablet form, but it is so toxic that about 35 per cent of patients have suffered side effects bad enough to make them stop the treatment.[2] In fact, gold is considered so dangerous that many specialists are turning to methotrexate as a safer option.[3]

Common among the side effects of most SAARDs are nausea, vomiting, abdominal pain and diarrhoea. Yet, even after suffering these reactions, the patient may be no better off. Benefits have been either observational or studied for only a short period of time. One double-blind study to test the second-line treatments against a placebo among 3,439 arthritis patients concluded that the benefits of the drugs were uncertain.[4]

Lack of research into long-term effects means that the patient has to play a game of Russian roulette to discover whether he or she will develop symptoms worse than their original condition. Fortunately, with gold treatment at least, an intolerance can usually be quickly spotted when the patient develops mouth sores or rashes.

Specialists don't understand how SAARDs work – if and when they do – but accept that they can be highly toxic and even life-threatening.[5] The overall impression is a stumble in the dark. As two American rheumatologists, Joseph Cash and John Klippel, concluded: 'substantial advances in the drug treatment of rheumatoid arthritis will require a much better understanding of the processes that propagate the disease and, ultimately, the identification of the factors that cause it'.[6]

Gold

The traditional and favoured SAARD, gold has even been described by some rheumatologists as the 'gold standard', a surprising title for a highly toxic treatment that can lead to fatal bone marrow suppression.[7]

Although gold has been in use as a treatment for arthritis since the 1920s, there has never been a long-term trial to test for reactions.

However, even over the short term, more than a third of patients find the side effects intolerable and stop treatment.[8]

Gold became the treatment of choice only because researchers misunderstood the causes of arthritis. German bacteriologist Robert Koch had shown that gold and other heavy metals could fight tuberculosis and other infectious diseases. As it was believed that arthritis was an infection, the theory was that gold could treat it.

Gold can be administered either as an injection, which was formerly the most common course, or in tablet form. The usual dose by injection is 50mg a week for 18 months, although the patient needs to be monitored carefully for early side effects, such as skin rash and mouth sores.

More serious adverse effects include kidney problems and bone marrow suppression. It is because of these concerns that gold in tablet form was developed.

Methotrexate

Methotrexate is fast becoming the most popular second-line therapy in the USA, as it has been found to be less toxic than gold in one Scottish study, an astonishing discovery for a powerful drug developed to treat cancer. In that study, average weekly dosages were 10mg/week and 1,460mg/week for methotrexate and gold, respectively.[9] The usual dose is 5–15mg a week, and improvement has been noted in 30–70 per cent of patients.[10]

However, the typical side effects of stomach complaints, nausea and anorexia can worsen dramatically if the dose is increased or the drug mixed with another. In the wrong hands, methotrexate is a potential killer, causing liver and kidney damage, lung disease and bone marrow suppression. Not surprisingly, the *Physicians' Desk Reference* reports deaths among arthritis patients taking the drug. The *PDR* stresses that the drug should be given only by 'physicians whose knowledge and experience includes the use of antimetabolite [the term refers to substances that fundamentally change the body's metabolism] therapy'.

This already powerful drug can form a lethal cocktail when taken with other drugs. Some rheumatologists are combining methotrexate with NSAIDs, which, on their own, account for thousands of deaths in Britain every year. Damage to the liver and lungs has been reported.[11]

It's long been known that methotrexate is a potential killer. Back in the 1990s, the National Patient Safety Agency announced that methotrexate, used for both arthritis and psoriasis, had led to 25 deaths and 26 cases of serious harm over a period of 10 years. Around the same time, reports came in about liver and kidney damage, lung disease and bone marrow suppression.[12] And researchers have warned of death among arthritis patients taking high doses, especially when taken daily instead of weekly.[13]

Sulphasalazine

Sulphasalazine belongs to the family of cytotoxic drugs that block the growth of cells. Serious side effects include bone marrow suppression, an increased risk of infection, infertility, cancer and defects in the embryo.[14] The drug was originally developed to treat ulcerative colitis and Crohn's disease. Its beneficial effects can be swift, usually apparent within two to three months.[15] In one study, a daily 2g dose achieved partial or complete remission from arthritis symptoms in 30 out of 59 patients.[16]

However, other studies show that, while sulphasalazine is better than a placebo, it has 'significant side effects' and is 'similar in efficacy to gold, but with lesser and milder toxicity'.[17]

Penicillamine

As the name suggests, penicillamine is a component of penicillin, originally developed to treat Wilson's disease (copper accumulation in the liver). For arthritis, the daily maintenance dose can be as high as 750mg, although the patient is usually started with 125–250mg to test for adverse reactions.

Common side effects include a skin rash, mouth ulcers and a loss of taste; a more serious reaction is skin eruptions, in which case the treatment should be stopped immediately. The blood disorder thrombocytopenia is common and can be severe.[18]

Chloroquine/hydroxychloroquine

These are antimalarial drugs that, through trial and error, have been found to have some beneficial effects on rheumatoid arthritis. They were used to treat a number of conditions after World War Two.

A common side effect is visual impairment that may even lead to blindness. The drugs may cause lesions in the eye with doses greater than 6mg a day.[19] Other effects include tinnitus, insomnia, hyperactivity and anaemia.

Cyclosporin

This immunosuppressant, originally developed to stop the body from rejecting a transplanted organ, has become another current 'flavour of the month' in medicine, used to treat every disease doctors otherwise don't know how to manage. It acts by reducing numbers of the immune system T cells, and should be used in treating rheumatoid arthritis only when the condition is life-threatening.

Other immunosuppressants that may be recommended are azathioprine and cyclophosphamide, both of which come with the same high risks. Common side effects are kidney dysfunction, high blood pressure and stomach problems.

Leflunomide

Leflunomide, a pyrimidine synthesis inhibitor, works by inhibiting an enzyme involved in the synthesis of a protein on the membrane of the mitochondria – the 'energy power pack' – of cells. This drug has been linked to six times more cases of fatal liver toxicity and 13 times more reports of hypertension than methotrexate, even though five times more prescriptions had been written for methotrexate. Marketed as Arava, leflunomide, which treats rheumatoid arthritis, has been linked to 12 deaths in the USA alone. The FDA has received at least 130 reports of severe liver toxicity from people taking the drug since it hit the market in 1998. Of these, 56 were treated in hospital and 12 died. Two of those who died were in their 20s.

Similar reactions to leflunomide have been reported in Europe, and the European Agency for the Evaluation of Medicinal Products issued an urgent warning to patients and doctors about the drug's toxicity after learning of 296 cases, 129 of which were serious, including liver failure. Public Citizen, a consumer watchdog group, petitioned the FDA to remove the drug from the marketplace. The drug was also linked to 12 cases of Stevens-Johnson syndrome (SJS), a serious systemic skin condition – an adverse reaction not seen with methotrexate.

Other side effects of leflunomide include diarrhoea, nausea, vomiting and anorexia, headache, dizziness, hair loss, eczema, dry skin, jaundice, anxiety, ruptured tendons and anaemia.

The link with possibly fatal liver toxicity was suspected at the time of licensing. Nevertheless, efforts to get the drug banned failed because an advisory panel to the FDA recommended that its benefits outweigh its 'rare' side effects.

TNF blockers

TNF blockers, which include Amgen and Wyeth's Enbrel, Abbott's Humira and Centocor's Remicade, are biologically engineered to relieve the worst and most painful symptoms of several forms of arthritis. Also called 'biological response modifiers', TNF blockers curtail the overproduction of TNF, an inflammation-regulating protein (TNF-alpha) that medical scientists believe is behind the inflammatory response seen in rheumatoid arthritis and other autoimmune disorders. As with many other drugs, TNF blockers act indiscriminately, crushing the immune response against any foreign agents TNF plays a major part in dealing with.[20]

Not long after the development and release of TNF blockers on the market, an FDA advisory panel met to determine whether they were behind some 170 cases of lymphoma that occurred among users of these drugs over a five-year period. The advisory panel issued several stiff warnings about these products, and the FDA asked manufacturer Centocor, a subsidiary of Johnson & Johnson, to revise its warnings in the prescribing information for bestselling arthritis TNF-blocking drug Remicade (also used to treat Crohn's disease), following evidence that it may cause cancer.

In more recent studies of all TNF-blocking agents, patients taking these drugs for arthritis were found to have three times the incidence of lymphoma than was usual among arthritis patients. Centocor itself admitted that in all its controlled trials their drug had a six-times higher incidence of this cancer than expected. Those most at risk included those with Crohn's disease and RA – the very population being prescribed the drug, many of whom were also frequently taking immunosuppressant drugs at the same time.

The FDA has advised all manufacturers producing TNF-blocking drugs to add to their product information a 'black box' warning (which the agency uses to highlight a drug's adverse effects) about the drug's potential to cause malignancy. The black box warning was a huge blow for companies such as Remicade's manufacturer Centocor. Remicade, a synthetically bio-engineered antibody (infliximab), was a top-selling intravenous drug in 2003, with sales of $1.5 billion in the USA alone. This drug can cause potentially fatal blood conditions such as leukopenia, neutropenia and pancytopenia (where the number of white blood cells capable of fighting infection is radically decreased), and inflammation and thickening of blood vessels. So far, there have been a number of deaths among people taking Remicade in combination with other drugs worldwide, although the FDA says it can't prove a direct causal link. Remicade is also implicated in numerous cases of pericardial effusion (fluid in the heart tissue).

Humira (adalimumab), a TNF blocker manufactured by Abbott Laboratories, is used to reduce symptoms in patients with moderate-to-severe rheumatoid arthritis, as well as to prevent bone damage and improve physical functioning in patients who haven't responded well to any other arthritis medication. Usually administered by injection every two weeks, Humira is also used to treat juvenile arthritis, psoriatic arthritis, ankylosing spondylitis and plaque psoriasis, and is also prescribed in the treatment of Crohn's disease.

Like etanercept (Enbrel) and infliximab (Remicade), it's associated with numerous dangerous side effects – specifically anaphylactic reactions and serious blood disorders such as pancytopenia and aplastic anaemia. And again like Enbrel and Remicade, Humira is also linked to an increased rate of tuberculosis (TB), serious fungal infections (endemic mycoses) and intracellular bacterial infections, even when used only for short periods of time.[21]

Previously, Humira's side effect profile and immunosuppressant action limited its use for only moderate-to-severe cases of RA in adults who failed to respond to other DMARDs. But now it's indicated as a go-to drug against all cases of RA, and its approval for ankylosing spondylitis (arthritis of the spine) is not far off.[22]

As for Humira's use for psoriatic arthritis, paradoxical effects have been reported. In one instance, five patients developed psoriatic skin lesions six to nine months after starting TNF-blocker drugs such as Humira. The lesions disappeared with topical treatment or on discontinuing the drug treatment.[23]

Some researchers question Humira's efficacy altogether, as placebo-controlled trials suggest that it's only moderately effective on its own, and that there's no point in continuing the drug for more than three months if it hasn't worked by then. The best results have been achieved in combination with another drug such as methotrexate, which of course has its own raft of side effects, including depressed bone marrow function.[24]

One of the most harmful side effects of TNF blockers is that they have contributed to the resurgence in tuberculosis, since they damage pro-inflammatory agents that nevertheless help to maintain TB in the latent phase. Anti-TNF medications appear to reactivate latent TB. They also disrupt calcified lung tissue containing live but dormant *Mycobacterium tuberculosis*, the bacteria that causes TB.[25]

So far several hundreds of cases of TB, in the lungs and in other organs, many of them fatal, have been associated with TNF-blocking agents.[26] The brain, lymph nodes and digestive tract may be involved, and there's even been a case of tonsillar TB in a 61-year-old RA patient after eight months of Humira treatment.[27]

Neither the FDA nor the various pharmaceutical manufacturers of this class of drugs are certain whether or not they reactivate latent tubercular infection or actually cause new infection. Nevertheless, Wyeth Pharmaceuticals, which makes Enbrel, has admitted that some patients who tested negative for latent TB prior to receiving the drug went on to develop active TB later.

In its own information leaflets, Wyeth also claims that as many as 7 per cent of patients given Enbrel with another drug for six months went on to develop serious infections, including bacterial pneumonia, cellulitis (bacterial skin infection), pulmonary fibrosis and fatal pneumonia. One patient with pulmonary fibrosis and pneumonia died as a result of respiratory failure. Of all the patients given the drug, nearly twice as many will go on to develop upper respiratory infections as those given a placebo.

Besides lung infections, TNF blockers have been found to cause viral, bacterial, fungal and protozoal infections in all organs, whether taking the drug alone or with other immunosuppressants. Those particularly susceptible include diabetics, those at risk of recurrent infections or those with open wounds. And as these types of infections have been implicated in arthritis, this raises the question of whether the 'cure' is actually worse than the disease.

There are also questions about TNF blockers' long-term effects, including documented side effects such as congestive heart failure, a lupus-like syndrome, lymphomas, blood-cell deficiencies and a multiple-sclerosis type of neurological disease. The most common, 'non-threatening' side effects are injection site reactions, and a skin rash is sometimes seen.[28]

A cancer connection in children

At present, the FDA is especially concerned about the possible association between TNF blockers and lymphoma and other cancers in children and young adults after receiving around 30 reports of cancer in this population group between 1998 and April 2008.

The reports describe the development of cancer in children and young adults taking TNF blockers when they were under 18 years of age. Approximately half the cancers were lymphomas

– both Hodgkin's and non-Hodgkin's types. The FDA has also received reports of other cancers in children and young adults, including leukaemia, melanoma and organ cancers, while taking the TNF blockers.

All this, and yet there's no real evidence that more is better when it comes to second-line treatments. Researchers carried out a meta-analysis of 101 studies of people with rheumatoid arthritis, which either compared a number of DMARDS against TNF-blocking drugs head to head or followed at least 100 patients on a single DMARD for 12 weeks or more. The researchers concluded that, on their own, all the tested drugs have a similar therapeutic effect, along with similar side effects. Combining two drugs seemed to help a little, especially when just one of the drugs on its own was having little effect, but there was insufficient data to assert categorically that this was the better approach.[29]

Dangers of TNF blockers

TNF blockers can cause:

⇨ Susceptibility to infection and lymphomas

⇨ Lupus-like symptoms

⇨ Abdominal pain

⇨ Swelling in the extremities

⇨ Stomach upset

⇨ Respiratory disorders

⇨ Sinusitis

⇨ Rhinitis

⇨ Nausea

⇨ Vomiting

⇨ Sore throat

⇨ Mouth ulcers

⇨ Coughing

⇨ Hair loss

⇨ Loss of strength

Steroids

After the immunosuppressants, steroids are the most controversial – and possibly most damaging – treatments available for arthritis. Steroid overuse in the 1950s for arthritis and the horrors resulting from this have put paid to this treatment among those with long enough memories. The Medical Research Council trial in 1960 concluded that the risks outweighed any benefits.

Steroids – such as cortisol, cortisone, prednisone and dexamethasone – are the oldest group of anti-arthritis drugs. Injected in large doses, they can reduce inflammation of the joints, and so reduce the pain of arthritis. They are closely related to cortisol, a hormone produced by the adrenal gland that helps the body to regulate its salt and water balance, as well as the metabolism of carbohydrates, fat and proteins. Steroids block the production of such chemical substances as prostoglandins, which trigger allergic and inflammatory reactions

– since in arthritis conditions, these reactions occur in an out-of-control cascade. Steroids also interfere with certain functions of the immune system and the production of white blood cells designed to destroy foreign bodies and infection.

Unfortunately, this interference with white blood-cell function creates numerous side effects as well as an increased susceptibility to infection.

Most doctors work on the assumption that steroids are safe if taken over a short period of time, and regularly prescribe them for any inflammatory or allergic reaction including skin and back problems, asthma, eczema, arthritis and bowel problems such as ulcerative colitis. Steroids have even been used as a replacement for baby's gripe water. The shots usually include a local anaesthetic and in many cases can be administered in your doctor's surgery. But research suggests that serious adverse reactions can happen right after treatment has started.

The side effects of steroids are many and various, including, in the words of a 2013 study, 'growth retardation in children, immunosuppression, hypertension, hyperglycaemia, inhibition of wound repair, osteoporosis, metabolic disturbances, glaucoma, and cataracts' and 'psychiatric' effects such as 'catatonia, decreased concentration, agitation, insomnia, and abnormal behaviours'.[30]

As one report concluded, 'The anti-inflammatory effects of corticosteroids cannot be separated from their metabolic effects',[31] which means that these drugs affect all cells of the body.

Long-term use of steroids can lead to loss of bone mineral density and can cause spinal fractures. One major study found that patients in the Netherlands suffered permanent damage to the bone mineral density in the lower spine after just 20 weeks of taking prednisone for rheumatoid arthritis.[32] In another case, nine-year-old Lexi McConnell was dead within five weeks of starting steroids to treat toxoplasmosis in the eye. Steroids can also stop the pituitary glands from producing ACTH, a hormone that regulates the adrenals, needed by the body during stress and to fight infections. Adrenal suppression (and therefore not enough cortisol) due to high-dose inhaled corticosteroids can even result in death, especially in children with asthma.[33] Steroids can even cause bone cell death (osteonecrosis), requiring complete joint replacement in some cases.[34]

Oral steroid use increases the risk of acute pancreatitis by 70 per cent, which can be a life-threatening problem in up to 20 per cent of cases.[35]

||||||||||||||||||||||||||||||||||||||||||||||

Chapter 4

OPERATIONS FOR ARTHRITIS

There's no doubt that replacing the cartilage in hip or knee joints that's been worn away by osteoarthritis with an artificial joint has transformed the life of many older people who would otherwise be confined to a wheelchair.

Hip replacement is now thought to be the most common form of surgery in the UK. However, there's a catch – and it's not just the long waiting lists for the procedure on the NHS. You might not think such a commonly performed operation could turn into a walking time-bomb, but varying surgical standards and the use of unproven materials are being blamed for hip replacements wearing out, and a wide range of life-threatening side effects – from chronic infection to cancer and thrombosis.

Advancements in surgical diagnosis, such as arthroscopy, whereby a fibre optic lens is inserted into a joint to help diagnose the damage and assist doctors in making recommendations, are far less invasive than the old-style 'let's cut you open and see' approach. Even so, having surgery is certainly not a choice for anyone to make lightly. A 2013 study conducted as part of the series 'When Health Care Makes You Sick' by *USA Today* found that unnecessary surgeries might account for 10 to 20 per cent of all operations – especially in the medical specialities.

Arthroscopic surgery

Arthroscopic surgery is the most common surgical procedure orthopaedic surgeons use to visualize, diagnose and treat problems inside a joint. It's most frequently performed on the knee and shoulder joints, less commonly on the hip, wrist, elbow and ankle. The reason the knee and shoulder are the most usually arthroscoped joints is that they are large enough for surgeons to manoeuvre the instruments around, and thus are more accessible to arthroscopic treatment.

In an arthroscopic examination, an orthopaedic surgeon makes a small incision and inserts a small camera lens and fibre-optic lighting system inside the joint to magnify and illuminate the cartilage and ligaments and other structures, displaying them for the doctor on a TV or computer monitor.

Even if the doctor does nothing but an exploration, after this type of surgery it takes several weeks for the joint to recover fully. A specific activity and rehabilitation programme may be suggested to speed recovery and protect future joint function.

A synovectomy commonly accompanies arthroscopy. This is performed to partially or completely remove the synovial membrane of a joint, with the aim of reducing the pain and swelling of rheumatoid arthritis and slowing the destruction of joints. However, this is usually a temporary measure: the synovium often grows back several years after surgery and the problem can happen again.

In mild cases, shoulder (glenohumeral) arthritis may be treated with arthroscopy. During the procedure the inside of the joint is debrided (cleaned out). But again, further surgery is often required.

Arthroscopic joint debridement is a minimally invasive surgery to the lining of joints, including the ankle joint (an area commonly affected by arthritis), where areas of loose, 'mechanically redundant' cartilage and inflamed tissue (synovitis) are removed from the joint. Loose fragments of bone within the joint and even bone 'spurs' (osteophytes) at the front of the joint can also be removed. Usually this procedure is useful only for patients with mild-to-moderate arthritis where the symptoms are not too severe and sufficient joint space shows up on X-rays.

Arthroscopic surgery is carried out around 650,000 times a year in the USA alone, and is the last option before knee replacement surgery for osteoarthritis sufferers. Around half the patients say they feel a big improvement in pain levels and movement afterwards,[1] although there's never been evidence to suggest the procedure either cures or arrests the osteoarthritic process. In fact, in a study of 180 patients, researchers discovered that surgery is no better than a placebo. In other words, patients who underwent 'dummy' surgery, during which nothing was done to them, reported the same benefits as those who'd received the full arthroscopic treatment.[2]

Joint replacement surgery

Joint replacement, or 'arthroplasty' as doctors term it, is justifiably regarded as miracle surgery. In the case of a hip replacement, the ball-and-socket joint of the hip, worn away by osteoarthritis, is replaced with an artificial joint made of a mix of metal and polyethylene (plastic).

During surgery, the surgeon removes the top of the femur (thigh bone) and replaces it with a metal ball attached to a long metal stem that is inserted into the hollow middle of the thigh bone. He then replaces the worn cup-like socket (acetabulum) of the pelvic bone – into which the rounded head of the femur fits, making up the hip joint – with a plastic or metal cup with a plastic lining.

These days, surgeons often use cementless metal balls in the thigh bone, relying instead on the porous metal titanium to adhere to the bone, and manufacturers are also experimenting with metal-on-metal components (a mix of cobalt–chromium and molybdenum alloys) to avoid the wear and tear seen with plastic components in the hope that these types of replacement hips will last longer and so be of use in younger patients.

The operation has become routine for most orthopaedic surgeons, who boast success rates of 98 per cent. Indeed, the age at which patients are recommended for such a hip op is spiralling downward: in one recent study, the median patient's age was 48.

Total hip replacement, invented in 1962 by English country orthopaedic surgeon John Charnley, has gone on to become one of the great surgical feats of the last century. It's now estimated that 10 per cent of people over 65 have a hip replacement, making it the most common form of surgery in the UK.

The fine print

However, that 98 per cent success rate refers to the number of patients who are wheeled out of surgery alive with the new hip intact. It doesn't cover the casualties that occur subsequently, which can range from death to a permanent abnormal gait or lifelong illness. Particularly if you're young, you should know about these possible side effects before you agree to the operation.

If an operation goes wrong, you could:

Die within a few months: According to one study, the death rate after just one month was 0.29 per cent, or 290 deaths out of every 100,000 operations. A review of the Norwegian Arthroplasty Register found a mortality rate of around 15 per cent (6,201 deaths out of 39,543 patients); of those deaths, 323 (about 5 per cent) occurred within the first 60 days after surgery. Overall, there was a 39 per cent greater mortality than expected in the general population.[3]

Develop venous thrombosis: This is a major risk after hip and knee surgery. Non-fatal venous thrombo-embolism after surgery – when a clot dislodges from a leg or lung vein and causes blockage in another part of the circulation, often an artery going to your lungs – occurs in one in 32 patients; fatal pulmonary embolism befalls around one in 100 patients. Those having knee replacement surgery had double the risk of deep vein thrombosis in the week following surgery than those undergoing hip replacement.[4]

Suffer from chip-off debris, resulting in autoimmune disease: The friction caused by the metal ball rubbing against the polyethylene socket lining causes small plastic or metal particles to flake off.

The body's immune system sees these particles as foreign invaders and attacks them – and because the particles typically settle near the implant, the immune system will also attack the surrounding bone (osteolysis). As bone loss occurs, the hip implant loosens and begins to function improperly. Osteolysis is considered the number one reason for implant failure and the need for a repeat operation.

A group of researchers called the Bristol Wear Debris Analysis Team discovered that in some cases particles of metals like nickel, chrome, titanium and cobalt, and even the bone cement (which contains hard ceramic particles of barium sulphate or zirconia), had worked their way from the hip joint to the liver, spleen, lymph nodes and bone marrow.

The greatest particle migrations were seen in those whose joint replacements were loose and worn, where the main problem was the matte coating used in the joint. In one patient, the level of cobalt found in the bone marrow was several thousands of times higher than normal.[5] In the case of a Frenchman complaining of weight loss and fatigue, wear debris had travelled into his spleen and liver eight years after surgery.[6]

Have the hip dislocate: This can happen either immediately or later, requiring repeat surgery.

End up with one leg appreciably shorter than the other: If the joint surface needs to be fused, as happens after some failed operations, you can end up with one leg as much as two to three inches shorter than the other.[7] This may happen in any case as many surgeons, to stabilize the hip so that it won't dislocate, deliberately make one leg a bit longer or shorter.

Eventually need a replacement: In other words, have the artificial hip replaced with a new one. After 10–15 years, the hip will be worn and in need of 'revision' – a replacement hip joint. This is a far more formidable operation, requiring the removal of more bone and tissue, and has a far lower success rate. If you're under 60, you face having to undergo several more revision operations in your lifetime.

Suffer damage to the sciatic nerve: This is the large nerve that runs down your leg. Repair neurosurgery has a poor success rate.

Develop cancer near the implant site: One study found associations between cancer of the lymph nodes and leukaemia, and hip replacement.[8] In a recent survey of 116,727 hip-replacement patients in Sweden, there was evidence of increased risks of melanoma (skin cancer), prostate cancer, multiple myeloma (bone marrow cancer) and bladder cancer.[9]

Safer surgery

Do whatever you can to avoid surgery by treating your osteoarthritis holistically (*see Chapters 7–10*). Think twice about going under the knife, especially if you are under 60: if you do have surgery below this age, it's extremely likely that you'll need a revision in your lifetime. But if you must have joint replacement surgery:

Use the cementless variety of ball-and-socket replacement if your bones are strong.

Insist on a hospital and a surgeon with a long and successful track record in performing this particular operation.

Opt for tried-and-tested materials. At the last count, there were more than 60 brands of artificial hips. In a 1998 health technology assessment of all research on the various hip brands, the lowest revision rates were seen with the Exeter, Lubinus and Charnley prostheses. In fact, in one study, two-thirds of Charnley prostheses, among the oldest and best-tested models, were still operational after 25 years.[10] Another good performer is the Stanmore.[11] More recently, metal-on-metal stemmed prostheses had higher failure rates than other types, and using them in combination with large head sizes led to particularly high rates of revision surgery in men and women up to 6 per cent of the time. The metal-on-polyethylene devices with 28mm head sizes had the lowest revision rates for women (1.6 per cent at five years), while the ceramic-on-ceramic with larger (40mm) head sizes proved the best option for men over 60 (with revision rates of 2 per cent at five years).[12]

Among the cementless varieties, the AML Total Hip Replacement is the most widely used model in the world. The lowest wear rate, as of the year 2000, was with metal-on-metal (alumina-on-alumina).[13] More recent research suggests that devices using highly cross-linked polyethylene cup liners are the most durable and cost-effective for most patients.[14]

Avoid these products: hip prostheses made from zirconia ceramic, hydroxyapatite(HA)-coated total hip replacements with a thin polyethylene inlay, and the W Hex Loc cementless hip socket.[15]

Knee replacement surgery

Besides hips, other joints such as the knees, shoulders, elbows, ankles and knuckles may also be replaced. Like hip replacement surgery, knee replacement surgery is the last resort when pain and immobility have become too great, and, like hip replacement, is performed under a general anaesthesia. In the operation, the surgeon removes the damaged cartilage (the soft lining of the joint), plus a small amount of bone. An artificial joint made of metal and polyethylene is cemented into place. A patient with no complications usually spends around five days in hospital, and a month recuperating at home, returning to normal activity over the course of two to three months.

The medical research paints a glowing picture of knee replacement, claiming that 95 per cent of knee operations using cement are successful (that is, have no complications) for at least a decade. According to a review of 130 studies,[16] 89 per cent of knee replacements have a good outcome over an average follow-up period of more than four years, and the majority of knee replacements remain functional for at least 10 years.

However, that sterling track record refers simply to knee replacements that 'take', and omits all the problems that could occur. The above-mentioned review came up with an overall complication rate of 18 per cent among those studies that reported on complications, including superficial infections, deep infections, pulmonary embolism (a blockage in a vein in the lung), deep venous thrombosis (blood clot in a vein) and nerve damage to a limb.

There are also admittedly small risks of other nerve or artery injury, permanent foot injury or, the worst-case scenario, loss of the limb. Complications can mean the patient is in hospital for a longer period of time and can even be subject to repeated operations.

Since the 1980s, medical technology firms have been trying to fix artificial knees biologically to bone via little metal beads or mesh.

But these 'uncemented porous-coated knee replacements' haven't been as successful as the cemented joints. According to one of many studies demonstrating this in the prestigious *Journal of Bone and Joint Surgery* (July 1991), out of 96 patients undergoing 108 replacements, about a fifth had failed owing to problems with the lower leg component. After seven years, more than half of these replacements were recommended for revision.[17]

As with hip replacements, it's important to understand that the knee will never be as good as new. Although such an operation may (though it may not) end chronic pain and enable you to move, doctors recognize that nothing artificial can match the versatility of a human joint. As with hip replacements, you need to hold off such an operation for as long as you can, because an artificial knee will only last about a decade before becoming fatigued; and at that point, you'll have to replace the knee replacement – a more formidable operation, with far more bone loss, removal of scarred tissue and a far lower success rate.

Too many surgeries

Perhaps dazzled by the success rate, doctors are too quick to replace knees. A new study has discovered that approximately one third of knee replacements in arthritis sufferers shouldn't have happened in the first place. And the need for such surgery was inconclusive in a further 22 per cent of cases, which suggests that potentially more than half of all total knee replacement procedures are dubious. Since approximately 600,000 knee replacements are done in the USA every year, more than 200,000 were unnecessary if these research findings are to be believed.[18]

Only 44 per cent of procedures were fully justified, say researchers from the Virginia Commonwealth University in the USA, after analysing 205 cases of total knee replacements.

All this suggests that anyone suffering with debilitating pain from arthritis (either rheumatoid or osteoarthritis) should consider knee replacement only if they've tried non-surgical approaches and failed.

Other types of surgery for arthritis

Ankle fusion is called arthrodesis of the ankle: the bones of the ankle joint are fused together, fixing the ankle completely in one position. Currently considered the gold-standard surgical treatment for managing patients with advanced ankle arthritis, its main objective is to relieve pain and improve overall function.[19] However, the procedure is technically complicated, often involving metal plates and screws to keep the bones in place, and the results vary widely.[20] There's also a high incidence of complications, so you'd be right to think twice before going under the knife.

One of the most common adverse consequences of ankle arthrodesis is non-union, when the bones fail to fuse, with reported fail rates as high as 40 per cent.[21] However, one review claims that these rates are steadily declining with the development of more advanced techniques.[22]

Nevertheless, if arthrodesis fails, a further operation is usually required and, if unsuccessful, may in some cases lead to amputation.[23] Another problem with arthrodesis is that, to compensate for the lack of ankle movement, the other joints have to move much more, creating excess strain on those joints and, in the long run, more pain and disability. Indeed, one arthrodesis follow-up survey concluded bleakly: 'Although ankle arthrodesis may provide good early relief of pain, it is associated with premature deterioration of other joints of the foot and eventual arthritis, pain, and dysfunction.'[24]

Other studies report that ankle-fusion patients tend to develop pain and moderate to severe arthritis in the joints of the foot.[25] This suggests that arthrodesis merely shifts the problem from one set of joints to another.

If this isn't enough to put you off, there are a number of other risks from surgery to consider, including deep infection, mal-union (the bones fusing in an imperfect position), delayed healing of the wound, stress fracture, neurovascular injury and deep vein thrombosis.[26] You should also bear in mind that your gait will be permanently altered, and it's likely that you'll have to wear special footwear afterwards.[27]

One other surgical risk worth is noting. Early anterior cruciate ligament (ACL) surgery performed on a teenager after knee injury is being recognized as a likely cause of osteoarthritis in later life. A study has found that around 65 per cent of patients suffered from arthritis of the knee within 20 years of having the surgery.[28] If your teenager injures himself or herself playing sport and ends up with a ruptured ACL, consider a stem-cell procedure (*see Chapter 11*) or even just exercise rehabilitation with a fully qualified physiotherapist, with experience of rehabilitating people with unreconstructed ACLs. Many physios now recognize that it is possible develop enough muscle strength to compensate for not having a functioning ACL.

The bottom line is this: surgery can help elderly people regain mobility when there's no other alternative to a wheelchair. However, for everyone else, it makes sense to do everything possible to avoid going under the knife, because in many instances surgery is no better than a placebo.

Consider the work of Dr Bruce Moseley, a specialist in orthopaedics at the Baylor College of Medicine in Houston, who tested 180 patients with severe osteoarthritis of the knee, dividing them into three groups. One group was given arthroscopic lavage (which washes away degenerative tissue and debris with the aid of a little viewing tube). Another received another form of debridement (removal of fronds of joint material by sucking them out with a tiny vacuum system). The third group was given a sham operation: patients were surgically prepared, placed under anaesthesia and wheeled into the operating room; incisions were made in their knees, but no actual procedure was carried out.

Over the next two years, during which time none of the patients knew who'd received the real operations and who'd received the sham treatment, all three groups reported moderate improvement in pain and function. In fact, the placebo group reported better results than some who'd received the actual operation.[29] The mental expectation of healing was enough to marshal the body's healing mechanisms. The intention, brought about by the expectation of a successful operation, produced the physical improvements, not the surgery itself.

Part II

THE DIETARY APPROACH TO ARTHRITIS

Chapter 5

IT'S NOT OLD AGE, IT'S INFLAMMATION

Researchers at Stanford University have made an explosive discovery that threatens to kick away the central platform of osteoarthritis treatment. Doctors have long assumed that the disease is largely caused by traumatic injury or by mechanical problems of 'wear and tear', like a piece of worn-out machinery. But as the Stanford research suggests, the disease, and what appears to be mechanical wear, may in fact be largely driven by low-grade inflammation.

In 2011, associate professor of immunology and rheumatology William Robinson and his colleagues at Stanford carried out studies showing that osteoarthritic joint tissues contain larger than usual numbers of migratory inflammatory cells that secrete certain substances early on in the progression of the disease.

The presence of these substances triggers the 'complement cascade', a chain of molecular events that eventually escalates into an attack – mounted by the body's own defence systems (which are usually only deployed against invading micro-organisms) – against the joint itself.

Doctors have witnessed evidence of inflammation in the cells of osteoarthritis patients (albeit not nearly as much as in rheumatoid arthritis), but the Stanford team's discovery of a heightened number of inflammatory cells in the early stages of the disease, before it causes symptoms, suggests that inflammation could be its central 'driver'.

Such findings suggest that osteoarthritis, like rheumatoid arthritis, is in fact an autoimmune condition – whereby the body begins to attack itself. This would explain why osteoarthritis isn't simply a disease of the elderly but, in many instances, starts in a person's 40s.

Robinson and his team made use of sophisticated lab techniques to compare levels of proteins present in the joint fluid of osteoarthritis patients with protein levels in the joints of healthy, non-arthritic people. The team discovered an enhanced expression of genes that activate inflammatory proteins, a larger than normal number of proteins that accelerate the complement cascade and a smaller than normal number of proteins that act as a brake.

When the researchers examined how this process could lead to osteoarthritis in the joints of both animals and humans, they discovered a cluster of proteins called the 'membrane attack complex' (MAC), the nuclear weaponry of the complement system, which binds to cartilage-producing cells. Ordinarily the MAC reserves its might to punch holes in virus- or bacteria-infected cells, but binding instead to cartilage cells causes them to secrete more complement-cascade proteins, inflammatory chemicals and enzymes than usual.

This process ultimately destroys cartilage, while a breakdown product of this cartilage destruction called 'fibromodulin' keeps switching the complement system on, so creating a continuing cycle of destruction.

When the researchers examined the joints of animals that had developed arthritis, they found an association between the level of attack by the complement system and the level of functional impairment – the more active the complement system, the more abnormal the animal's gait.[1]

'This low-grade complement activation,' said Robinson, 'contributes to the development of degenerative diseases, including Alzheimer's disease and macular degeneration. Our results suggest that osteoarthritis can be added to this list.'[2]

Robinson considers the discovery a paradigm shift in the way medicine sees arthritis. The current medical view is that osteoarthritis is incurable, and the usual recommendations are to lose weight, exercise to increase muscle strength, and take numerous drugs to manage the pain and supposedly the inflammation too. The course of treatment is a tightrope walk between reducing pain and not bringing about a great deal of toxic effects on the heart and liver.

These relatively new findings have huge implications for how medicine deals with osteoarthritis. Rather than treating it as an inevitable part of growing old, the Stanford research suggests that an individual's lifestyle might be analysed to determine what's causing the chronic inflammation and what sorts of natural compounds might help lower it to inhibit progression of the cycle.

This represents the first laboratory confirmation of what many practitioners of functional medicine have found to be the case in clinical practice. Dr John Mansfield, author of *Arthritis: The Allergy Connection* (Chivers Press, 1991), who successfully treated several thousands of arthritis patients in the UK at his clinic in Surrey before recently retiring, believes that most forms of arthritis are 'environmentally induced' by an intolerance to food or certain environmental chemicals and that some 90 per cent of patients can be improved or fully cured just by making certain lifestyle changes.

What is inflammation?

Every 'itis' condition you've ever heard of – arthritis, bronchitis, gastritis, tonsillitis, neuritis – is an inflammation condition resulting from the body's natural attempt to induce healing by increasing blood and lymph flow carrying nutrients into a damaged or negatively affected area while also flushing harmful pathogens, irritants and damaged cells away from the site.

Characterized by swelling, heat, redness and pain, inflammation is fundamentally a healing immune system response to injury, toxins, allergy and infection. Initial inflammation conditions are called 'acute inflammation' (often frequently accompanied by acute pain), and are usually short-lived.

Chronic conditions such as joint pain are an inflammatory warning sign that something is systemically out of balance – that the body is struggling to maintain health in the face of an overwhelming assault of toxins, stressors and pro-inflammatory foods that are not only inhibiting normal healing, but also contributing to an ever-worsening cycle of pain and general disease, ultimately resulting in serious conditions such as cardiovascular disease and stroke.

An 'inflammation cascade' occurs when a tissue injury or pathogen of some sort (a virus, bacteria, parasite, fungal infection or allergens) triggers the creation of cytokines. These small proteins involved in cell signalling stimulate the production of cytotoxic (cell-destroying) chemicals – which is supposed to be part of the 'seek and destroy' mission of the immune system, and essential to the healing process.

When cascades get out of hand, the body ends up with an inflammation response that doesn't stop – as is the case with arthritis.

Arthritis and food allergies

The connection between food allergies/intolerance and arthritis was suggested over 60 years ago.[3] Early evidence was sparse but compelling. Finally, in the 1980s, a major study clearly showed that arthritis patients' symptoms improved on fasting, but worsened when they began to eat certain foods. The findings were supported by objective evidence from blood analyses.[4]

Increasingly, clinical ecologists (doctors who believe that food and lifestyle affect health) are concluding that arthritis is caused by food allergies or intolerances of certain environmental chemicals such as tobacco smoke, pesticides, perfume or even hairspray.

Medicine finally gave this theory a grudging nod when a Norwegian study published in *The Lancet* in the early 1990s revealed that patients with rheumatoid arthritis improved after 1) fasting, then

2) following a gluten-free vegan diet for three and a half months, after which 3) they were put on a lacto-vegetarian diet. The study group showed significant improvements in all areas measured, including number of tender and swollen joints, pain, stiffness, grip strength and even white blood-cell count. These benefits were still present a year after the study ended.[5]

Although food is the most common culprit, John Mansfield and others find that house dust mites and moulds, smoking and intestinal overgrowth of the yeast bug *Candida albican* can also bring on arthritic symptoms.

Doctors like Mansfield try to isolate the source of the food or chemical problem through skin prick tests (more useful for inhaled allergens than food ingredients, says Mansfield) and through elimination diets. The treatment is either to eliminate the offender from the diet, or to use a technique called 'provocation intradermal neutralization' or else enzyme-potentiated desensitization (EPD), the latter developed by Dr Len McEwen, formerly of the Department of Allergy at St Mary's Hospital, London. With the provocation neutralization techniques (favoured by Dr Mansfield as they have been subject to many more safety studies), a patient is given (by either injection or drops under the tongue) the dosage of the allergenic substance that 'turns off' the symptoms. This is discovered through a series of injections that 'provoke' allergenic responses.

It's been discovered that a small subcutaneous injection (that is, just under the skin) can protect a patient for the next two or three days should he or she eat the particular food to which he or she is intolerant. A cocktail of all the neutralizing doses of the foods to which the patient is sensitive, administered in a single injection about three times a week as a kind of 'vaccination', will enable the patient to eat normally. In the case of sublingual drops (that is, drops placed under the tongue), one drop will contain neutralizing doses for lots of different food allergens.

The same principles can be used to 'neutralize' reactions to inhaled allergens such as house dust, dust mites, moulds, animal furs and summer pollens. Mansfield reports that relief with inhaled allergen-neutralizing injections often starts within half an hour of the first injection and lasts for several days.

The great advantage of neutralization is that your diet or treatment is completely individualized. After two years of injections, the patient should become desensitized to the food in question and able to eat it without needing any more treatment.

The *dis*advantage is that, after weeks or months, the neutralizing levels can change, making the body resistant to higher and higher doses. This may make re-testing necessary, adding to the expense.

EPD

When the technique of enzyme-potentiated desensitization (EPD) was being developed, Dr McEwen used to scratch a large patch on the arm and place a large number of allergens in a container and strap it onto that area of skin on the arm. Now, EPD practitioners employ a large, intradermal injection of a blockbuster micro-dose of hundreds of allergens mixed with the enzyme glucuronidase (hence the name 'enzyme-potentiated desensitization'). The injection, which takes several months to work, is given at intervals over months. This therapy does not have the immediate relief of neutralization, but claims good responses over a period of months. The disadvantage with EPD is that we don't know the long-term effects.

Finding out what in your lifestyle is causing inflammation in your body is a matter of detective work. Consequently, you should carry out this investigation with a qualified and experienced nutritional practitioner, who can help you find the cause and choose from among a plethora of natural treatments that have been shown to work as well as, often even better than, drugs.

Do you have a food intolerance?

As more than 70 per cent of immune-system cells are found in the lining of the digestive tract, we're now recognizing a direct link between immune-system function and the gut. This means that the body's immune system is enormously affected by the foods we do or don't eat, or by the overall state of our digestive system. In recent years it's been discovered that some foods actually induce an inflammatory response and other foods shut it down.

We also know that inflammatory and autoimmune diseases such as arthritis have radically increased in direct proportion to the development and consumption of highly processed, wheat- and corn-based, sugar- and preservative-filled or genetically modified convenience foods. When the processed foods were introduced some 50 years ago, degenerative diseases such as arthritis, diabetes and cardiovascular disease were certainly not as widespread as they are today; and most processed foods are laden with the most common allergenic ingredients, as we'll soon discover.

Many integrative and nutritional doctors and naturopaths agree that osteoarthritis is often caused by food allergies or intolerances, and that a majority of arthritis patients are sensitive to foods in the nightshade, or *Solanaceae*, plant family. This food group includes white potatoes, eggplant (aubergine), sweet and hot peppers such as cayenne and paprika (not the black and white kind sprinkled on food), tomatoes and tobacco. The entire nightshade family contains many of the natural toxic chemicals of belladonna (deadly nightshade).[6] In a survey of 763 arthritis sufferers carried out by researchers from Rutgers University and the University of Florida, 73 per cent claimed to have responded positively to a diet eliminating nightshades; 28 per cent of the responses were so marked that 'immobilized joints became mobile' again, and "canes, walkers and wheelchairs were discarded'. When the survey was carried out again, this time of 434 responders, 68 reported various degrees of relief from arthritic symptoms; of the 52 per cent who were rigidly on the diet, 94 per cent reported 'complete or substantial relief'.[7]

The late Dr Collin H. Dong of San Francisco, himself a victim of arthritis, developed a 'caveman-type' diet to deal with his own crippling arthritis. Within a few months he was free of symptoms and able to return to playing golf.

The Dong diet was devised to avoid many of the most common allergens, including artificial ones, as well as meat, fruit (including tomatoes), dairy, vinegar and other acids, all varieties of pepper, hot spices, chocolate, dry-roasted nuts, all alcohol (particularly wine), carbonated soft drinks, and all additives, preservatives and chemicals, especially monosodium glutamate (MSG). Because it avoids meat, the diet is naturally high in fish, and fish oils are now widely recommended as good for arthritis patients.

Suspect an allergy if you have: weight issues (either over- or underweight), swelling of the hands, eyes, ankles or abdomen, excessive sweating, even with no exertion, constant fatigue despite adequate sleep, and a too rapid heart rate, especially after meals.

The 15 most common allergens

If you have arthritis, first suspect a food intolerance or allergy to one of the big 15:

⇨ Dairy (including animal milks, kefir and yoghurt, cheeses and butter)

⇨ Soya

⇨ Wheat

⇨ Gluten (a protein present in wheat, rye, some oats and barley)

⇨ Potatoes and other nightshades (tomatoes, peppers, aubergines and tobacco)

⇨ Beef

⇨ Refined sugar

⇨ Chocolate

⇨ Coffee

⇨ Corn

⇨ Eggs

⇨ Oranges

⇨ Pork

⇨ Tea

⇨ Yeast

A royal role for purines

Centuries ago physicians had no difficulty linking gout – known as 'the disease of kings' or the 'rich man's disease' because most patients developing gout were wealthy and obese – to a high consumption of alcohol, meats, sweets and seafood. These were foodstuffs only the rich could afford to consume, let alone in excess. As it turns out, the old-time belief in a dietary cause for gout was spot on. High consumption of organ meats, shellfish, anchovies, sardines, asparagus and mushrooms all contribute to gout because all these foods are high in purines – chemicals the body converts to uric acid, which builds up in the blood, leading to the formation of crystals in a joint, thereby causing pain and inflammation.

Today, other risk factors for gout include excessive alcohol consumption, especially beer and spirits, as well as certain illnesses and medications. People who suffer from hypertension, diabetes, kidney disease and SLE (lupus) are more vulnerable to gout, as are those who regularly take diuretics, low-dose aspirin (1–2g/day) and drugs commonly prescribed to organ transplant recipients such as cyclosporine.[8] An often overlooked cause of gout is lead poisoning,[9] caused by the kidneys failing to excrete excess lead effectively.

Are you overweight?

Carrying too much weight increases the load on joints and seems to be one major factor in the advancement of arthritis. But common targets for osteoarthritis in overweight people include not only the weight-bearing joints of the body, such as the knees, but the finger joints too, suggesting that the link between obesity and osteoarthritis is due to factors other than just biomechanical loading.

Researchers at the Department of Orthopaedic Surgery at Washington University School of Medicine in St Louis, Missouri, believe that fat tissue is a major source of pro-inflammatory mediators such as cytokines, chemokines and adipokines – metabolic factors known to have inflammation-boosting properties that help to 'orchestrate' the process of osteoarthritis.[10]

The obesity connection may have more to do with a patient's overall diet and lifestyle, and how they contribute to insulin resistance and metabolic imbalances – the so-called 'metabolic syndrome', which is connected with atherosclerosis, diabetes and other modern-day degenerative diseases, including Alzheimer's. The major contributors are too much sugar, processed foods and fried foods, which all release oxidizing free radicals into the system. These, in excess, can damage the tissues around joints.

A poor diet can also cause dysfunction in the mitochondria, the power packs of our body's cells, which supply the energy needed for cells to do their jobs.[11]

Do you have an imbalance of fatty acids?

Today's processed diets feature too much omega-6 fatty acids, known to lead to inflammation and, in turn, joint destruction, swelling and pain, and too little omega-3 fatty acids.

These fatty acids, stored in our body's fat cells, are essential because we can't manufacture them in our body and so must obtain them from our diet. They provide energy, and help to build cell membranes and other important substances in the body such as hormones. Our body requires both saturated fats (the type available from butter and coconut oil) and also unsaturated fats (present in olive and other plant oils and fish oil). Omega-6 fatty acids, available in sunflower and soya oil, are plentiful in most Western diets, because they are present in processed foods, but we're now beginning to understand that it's the omega-3 fatty acids that lower inflammation as it occurs with arthritis, and that high levels of omega-6 fatty acids can cause oxidative damage to our cell membranes.

Nevertheless, the American government still recommends high levels of omega-6 fatty acids. The recommendation of the National Institute of Medicine of the US National Academy of Science of a 10 to 1 ratio of omega-6 to omega-3 fatty acids is weighted too much towards omega-6: other countries, including the UK's Department of Health, suggest a 4:1, 3:1 or even a 1:1 ratio. Such a ratio is thought to be beneficial by reducing the risk of many chronic conditions such as hypertension, cardiovascular disease, diabetes, arthritis and cancer.[12]

A quick guide to fats

There are two types of fats: saturated fats and unsaturated fats, which differ only in the bond between the atoms, but have vastly different effects on the body.

Saturated fats, made from a bond of a single carbon atom, are mostly from animal foods, but are also found in tropical oils such as palm and coconut oils. The saturated fats in our diets are generally derived from four types: stearic (animal fat and chocolate); lauric (coconut oil); palmitic (palm oil, animal products and dairy); and myristic (coconut oil and dairy).

Unsaturated fats come in two forms: monounsaturated fats (with one double carbon bond between atoms) and polyunsaturated fats (two double bonds). **Monounsaturated** fats are found in olive and canola oils, cashews, peanuts, macadamia nuts, almonds and avocados. **Polyunsaturated** fats include omega-3 and omega-6 fatty acids, described separately below:

Omega-3 fatty acids come from fatty fish such as salmon, mackerel, herring, sardines, and also flaxseeds. They comprise alpha-linolenic acid (ALA), found in flaxseed, and eicosapentaenoic acid (EPA) and docosahexaenoic acid (DHA) (found in plankton and fatty fish).

Omega-6 fatty acids are found in corn, safflower, sunflower, soya bean and sesame oils. They include linoleic acid (LA) and gamma-linolenic acid (GLA), both of which are converted in the body into prostaglandins, which perform many vital bodily functions. The evidence now suggests that excess omega-6s bring about chronic inflammation in the body, leading to a plethora of diseases, including arthritis, while omega-3 fatty acids lower inflammation.

Trans fats are formed when an oil goes through a process called hydrogenation, which makes it more solid. This type of fat, known as hydrogenated fat, used for frying or as an ingredient in processed foods, has been shown to damage health and contribute to diseases like arthritis.

Are you sensitive to a chemical?

We live in a world where constant exposure to dangerous chemical agents and pollutants is the norm. Industrial chemicals are not tested for safety before they are put on the market. The US Environmental Protection Agency has required safety testing for only a tiny fraction of the 85,000 industrial chemicals currently on the market in shampoos, hairspray, lotions, sunscreens, laundry detergents, cleaning agents and other chemicals typically found around the house.

And so far only five substances – hexavalent chromium, dioxin, polychlorinated biphenyls, asbestos and chlorofluorocarbons – have been banned, and only then in certain instances and applications. Add radiation, carbon monoxide from road vehicles, particulates from diesel vehicles, the release of volatile organic compounds (VOCs) from synthetics used in furniture, paints and carpeting, and you begin to understand why the human body has become a battle ground of toxicity.

The late Dr Theron Randolph of Chicago, Illinois, who first developed the theory of chemical sensitivity, found that household gas, formaldehyde and the pesticides found in food supplies contributed to many cases of arthritis. Indeed, many of British allergy specialist Dr Mansfield's patients immediately improved or entirely resolved their symptoms just by switching from gas to electricity for cooking.

People living near airports who are regularly exposed to jet fuels are far more likely to develop arthritis than others, as are people who are sensitive to second-hand smoke, food chemicals, other pollutants in the air, and even hairspray and lipstick. Professor Michael Ehrenfeld from Tel Aviv University has long believed that environmental factors have a large part to play in determining who develops the disease. 'Most people think arthritis has to do with old age,' he has said, 'but this is false.'[13]

Breast implants and other silicone prostheses have been shown to promote antibodies, or allergic responses, to collagen, which then collect in susceptible tissues,[14] and this has been linked with joint swelling. In fact, some women have seen their arthritic symptoms disappear after having their implants removed.

Do you have a leaky gut?

Increased intestinal permeability (so-called 'leaky gut') leads to the absorption of incompletely digested proteins through the gut wall, and this has been linked to many diseases, including arthritis and joint problems.[15]

If you've been taking non-steroidal anti-inflammatory drugs (NSAIDs) over the long term, then you almost certainly have a leaky gut, as these drugs are known to cause it. Just two doses of aspirin or indomethacin can increase permeability in the gut wall by lowering levels of the protective fatty acid prostaglandin.[16]

Long-term NSAID use (typical with osteoarthritis sufferers) leaves the gut very inflamed and highly permeable[17] and so perpetuates the problem. Medications can also stimulate an overabundance of harmful bacteria, such as *Prevotella copri* bacteria, which seem to play a part in triggering arthritis. Research shows that rheumatoid arthritis sufferers have far higher levels of these bacteria in their gut, although whether this is a case of direct cause and effect has yet to be proven.[18]

Do you have nutritional deficiencies or excesses?

An overabundance of unhealthy substances such as breads, refined white sugar and unbalanced omega-6 fatty acids, or a lack of normal healthy foods, such as leafy green vegetables and healthy fats such as omega-3 fatty acids, all can lead to hormonal disturbances, a stressed immune system and chronic inflammation. Often nutritional deficiencies are tied to food allergies. For example, undetected gluten intolerance causes inflammatory damage to the lining of the gut, preventing nutritional absorption of certain foods.

Do you suffer from stress or emotional trauma?

Emotions trigger chemical releases in the body – in fact, the work of the late neuroscientist and pharmacologist Dr Candace Pert (author of *Molecules of Emotion*, Simon & Schuster, 1999) shows that every single emotion has a unique chemical signature created by peptides – or what she referred to as 'molecules of emotion'. Unrelieved anxiety and stress, for examples, raise adrenaline and cortisol levels in the body, which can lead to hormonal imbalance and ongoing chronic inflammation. If you've had prolonged stress or emotional upsets, consider using some of the 'mind–body' approaches offered in Chapter 12.

Free radicals and 'earthing'

One interesting hypothesis for the rise of unchecked inflammation is that it results from two factors working together: production of free radicals, combined with a lack of electromagnetic grounding with the Earth.

Processed foods, sugar, pollution and chemical toxins have been proven to stimulate the production in the body of highly damaging free radicals – atoms, molecules and ions that have unpaired electrons and thus a positive charge. These are highly reactive and bond with other substances in the body causing, among other things, oxidative stress and inflammation.

In the old days, dangerous positively charged free radicals in the body were mitigated by regular contact with the Earth, which holds a negative electromagnetic charge. Walking barefoot or in leather-soled shoes permitted an influx of negatively charged electrons into the body, which could resupply the unbalanced positively charged atoms, molecules and ions (free radicals) with a much-needed electron. But with the introduction of rubber-soled shoes and rubber-tyred vehicles, that changed.

Proponents of 'earthing' say the process can provide a natural antidote to free-radical activity, because the negatively charged electrons from the Earth are able once again to counteract the positively charged free radicals. To demonstrate the theory, William Amalu, president of the International Academy of Clinical Thermography, used thermographic imaging – by which an infrared camera displays changes in skin surface temperatures – to plot the healing of 20 patients suffering from a range of inflammatory conditions, including muscle strain, carpal tunnel syndrome and inflammatory joint problems.

The patients were earthed with either a conductive electrode patch, applied in Amalu's office during two to three half-hour treatments a week, or a grounded bed pad in their homes where they slept at night. Some patients experienced improvements after just one week – and the thermographic images supported their claims. In at least 12 cases, an 80 per cent improvement was registered by thermography. Images of all 20 patients can be found in the book *Earthing: The Most Important Health Discovery Ever?* by Clinton Ober, Stephen T. Sinatra and Martin Zucker.[19]

Chapter 6

THE SECRET CONNECTION: YOUR GUT

In 1992, after rediscovering a network of neurotransmitters in the gut that act in a similar way to ordinary neurons, Dr Michael Gershon, chairman of the department of anatomy and cell biology at New York-Presbyterian Hospital/Columbia University Medical Center, an expert in the new field of neurogastroenterology, christened this phenomenon 'the second brain'.

He and others have since found that the enteric nervous system, as it's technically known, consists of some 30 neurotransmitters and vast sheaths of neurons embedded all along the nine metres of our alimentary canal – 100 million of them in all, more than are present in either the spinal cord or peripheral nervous system. In fact, the self-same genes involved in the formation of synapses between neurons in the primary brain are also involved in the formation of synapses in this so-called 'gut brain'.

All manner of modern-day illnesses link back to disturbances in the digestive system, including joint and muscle pain, and even autoimmune diseases such as motor neurone disease and rheumatoid arthritis.

In preliminary studies, researchers from Columbia University Medical Center have even demonstrated that a hormone secreted from the enteric nervous system is able to regulate bone mass and counteract osteoporosis.

Dr Alan Ebringer of London's Middlesex Hospital has linked ankylosing spondylitis, a painful arthritic disease resulting in progressive stiffening of joints, with a type of bacteria that lives in the bowel and feeds off carbohydrate residues. Many patients have resolved their long-standing conditions simply by switching to a low-carb diet.

Work going on now at the University of California at Los Angeles is examining how the human biome – the trillions of bacteria residing in the gut – communicates with nervous-system cells, and how this affects our emotions and moods.

Factor in the state of the gut bacteria and their ability to communicate with the gut brain, and you begin to recognize how central digestion is to overcoming all manner of physical illness such as arthritis.

Russian biologist and Nobel laureate Élie Metchnikoff once remarked, 'Death begins in the colon,' and for good reason. There's no doubt that one of the major keys to a long and healthy life lies in your body's ability to digest properly.

It's your digestive system – your stomach and intestines – that does most of the work of turning what you eat into fuel and nourishment for your body. This is a highly complex affair, aided by a huge army of enzymes, acids, friendly bacteria and peptides. If anything is even slightly awry or the balance is off in some way, no amount of organic food or supplements will keep you healthy.

Bad-guy gut bacteria

More than two-thirds of IBS patients who regularly suffer from diarrhoea have bacterial overgrowth in the gut, as do nearly a third of IBS patients overall, say researchers from the Cedars-Sinai Medical Center in Los Angeles. With this condition, officially known as 'bacterial dysbiosis', the bacteria alter the metabolic and immune responses of the body, causing the immune system to turn against the normal gut flora.[1] According to research, this situation is an early complication of a 'leaky gut'.[2]

In addition to food intolerance, this phenomenon, as we have seen, can also be caused by even short-term use of non-steroidal anti-inflammatory drugs (NSAIDs).[3] Long-term use of such drugs can leave the gut very inflamed and highly permeable. Also, people with rheumatoid arthritis and osteoarthritis taking NSAIDs have been found to have increased levels of antibodies to *Clostridium perfringens* bacteria compared with osteoarthritis patients who aren't taking NSAIDs, leading to the conclusion that bacterial toxins are involved.[4]

Suspect this as the cause of your arthritis: if you have taken multiple courses of NSAIDs and antibiotics, and eat genetically modified (GM) foods and saturated milk fats, all of which may be responsible for many gut problems.

Those saturated, milk-derived fats – found in processed foods and confectionery – upset bacteria in the gut within six months of eating a diet high in them, say researchers from the University of Chicago. They also encourage proliferation of *Bilophila wadsworthia* bacteria in the gut, a microbe associated with inflammatory gut disorders.[5]

Diagnose this: by taking the Hydrogen and Methane Breath Test, which involves swallowing a carbohydrate and measuring bacterial fermentation of the carb through breath samples of hydrogen and methane. Biolab in London offers the test (*see address, page 95*).

Solve this: by taking the following supplements:

⇨ Vitamin D, as people suffering from gut problems are usually deficient in this vitamin

⇨ 25–50mg of zinc, 2–4mg of copper, 800mcg of folic acid and 800mcg of vitamin B12, all of which can help repair the gut; and check your iron status too

⇨ Supplements of homoeostatic soil organisms (HSOs), good-guy organisms found naturally in soil that were part of the human diet before 1930 – these have been shown to calm an inflamed gut

⇨ Bentonite, or hydrated aluminium silicate, which has the remarkable ability to get bacteria and viruses to stick to it – since bentonite is not absorbed, it passes through the colon, taking toxins with it

Too much fruit sugar

About a third of patients with gut issues like IBS have 'fructose malabsorption', or difficulty processing fructose – the type of sugar found in fruits, some vegetables, honey and high-fructose corn syrup – as it passes through the small intestine.[6]

Suspect this as the cause of your arthritis: if your gut discomfort gets worse after eating fruit.

Diagnose this: by taking a fructose intolerance test, another breath test measuring your capacity to absorb any sort of fructose.

Solve this: by limiting the amount of fruit sugar you eat. One Mayo Health System study in America found that 38 per cent of patients reduced their symptoms just by lowering their consumption of fruit sugars. In particular, children with previous diagnoses of abdominal pain caused by a functional bowel disorder respond well to a low-fructose diet.[7]

Also watch out for other fermentable, poorly absorbed carbohydrates like lactose (found in milk), fructans (found in wheat and onions) and sorbitol (a common sweetener),[8] and avoid amines (cheese, chocolate, citrus fruits, coffee and red wine) and food additives (benzoates, sulphites, nitrates and nitrites, and tartrazine and other artificial colours).

Low stomach acid

In many cases, people with gut problems produce too little or no stomach acid or digestive enzymes.

Suspect this as the cause of your arthritis: if you feel especially uncomfortable after eating.

Diagnose this: by getting a stomach-acid analysis done to discover how much gastric acid your stomach produces and also whether you've got enough pancreatic enzymes. Again, Biolab does these tests (*see page 95*).

Solve this: by supplementing your diet (according to directions on the label) with the stomach acid betaine hydrochloride (HCl plus pepsin) and pancreatic enzymes for at least 12 weeks. Taking 500mg of l-histadine can also improve gastric-acid production.

Avoid histamine blockers – or 'histamine H2-receptor antagonists' in medico-speak – sold over the counter to ease heartburn and acid reflux, as they do this by reducing levels of stomach acid.

A leaky gut wall

When working at peak condition, the lining of your small intestine acts like a smart sieve that allows only small particles of food – amino acids, carbs and essential fatty acids – to pass through it to reach your bloodstream and be transported to other cells in the body, while blocking other, larger food molecules and toxins or bacteria that might cause harm.

But if this tiny sieve is damaged in some way, a large number of these toxic substances are then able to breach the gut wall, triggering the production of antibodies that can lead to allergies, altering the bacterial composition of the gut and even allowing the overgrowth of fungal yeasts like *Candida*. A range of conditions – from ulcerative colitis, poor food absorption, Crohn's disease and IBS to malnutrition, skin complaints such as acne, psoriasis and dermatitis, and all manner of joint diseases – often hark back to having a sieve with holes that are just too big. In fact, people with joint pain have been found to have greater gut permeability and are more likely to respond to dietary measures.[9]

Suspect this as the cause of your arthritis: if you've been diagnosed with *Candida* infection but the treatment hasn't worked, or you've had radiotherapy, severe burns, periodic hives or dermatitis, or you suddenly seem to be reacting to an ever-increasing number of foods, particularly those from a range of different food groups.[10] Other causes are alcohol abuse, NSAIDs and chemotherapy.[11]

Also, a too permeable gut is often the result of a mouth full of amalgam fillings, after microscopic amounts of the mercury migrate to other places in the body, increasing allergic-type immune responses, according to animal and lab studies.[12]

Diagnose this: by taking a 'lactulose/mannitol challenge test'. Neither of these sugars is metabolized in the healthy gut and so should mostly be excreted in the urine after six hours. If the tests show more sugar than normal is taken up, you've got a gut that leaks.

(You can have this and other gut permeability tests done by Biolab in the UK or by Genova Diagnostics in Europe and the USA: *see page 95.*)

Solve this: by chewing your food thoroughly, as that releases epidermal growth factor (EGF), a polypeptide that stimulates the growth and repair of the small intestinal walls.[13] Make sure you include healthy fibre in your diet, which reduces your susceptibility to gut permeability.[14]

Healing your 'leaky' gut

Take supplements of any or all of the following and experiment to see which ones work best for you, or work with a qualified, experienced naturopath.

⇨ Probiotics have long been shown to improve gut permeability.[15] Choose strains containing *lactobacilli, bifidobacteria, Saccharomyces boulardii* and non-disease-causing strains of *Escherichia coli* and *streptococci*.

⇨ Vitamin A is necessary for the growth and repair of cells that line both the small and large intestines. Suggested supplement dosage: 10,000 International Units (IU).

⇨ Colostrum-derived supplements (available online at sites like www.biovea.com and www.myprotein.com) can improve the state of your gut lining and also encourage the growth of natural gut flora.

⇨ Glutamine, an amino acid essential for a sound gut wall, can repair the gut mucosal lining damage caused by chemotherapy and radiation.[16]

⇨ Glutathione (GSH) is an antioxidant, levels of which are often low in people with leaky gut syndrome. If you've got parasites too, don't supplement until you've cleared them first (*see page 91*).

⇨ Flavonoids like those found in milk thistle (*Silybum marianum*) and dandelion root (*Taraxacum officinale*), when taken before eating, can block allergic reactions that increase gut permeability.

⇨ Fish oils can protect the body against toxins produced in the gut and prevent injury to the gut wall caused by the second-line arthritis drug methotrexate.[17]

⇨ *Saccharomyces boulardii*, a gut-friendly yeast originally isolated from the skins of lychee fruits and used in 'yeast against yeast' treatment in France, can by itself reduce bouts of diarrhoea and colitis.[18]

⇨ The B vitamins and vitamins C and E, zinc, selenium, molybdenum, manganese and magnesium, all of which provide additional benefits towards healing the gut.

Parasites

About one in six of us is walking around with *Giardia lamblia*, a minuscule flagellated protozoan that causes severe fatigue and bowel disturbances, and one in 10 is infested with *Cryptosporidium*, another group of diarrhoea-causing protozoans.

These and other gut parasites such as *Blastocystis hominis* can cause vague gut symptoms that come and go or that mimic those of IBS. And now we also know that they may be linked to cases of rheumatoid arthritis.

In 1975, at the IXth International Chemotherapy Congress in London, the late microbiologist Roger Wyburn-Mason (MD, PhD) of the Mayo clinic and Yale University, announced the discovery of the presence of the protozoa species of *Naegleria* in cases of rheumatic disease: this may have been its cause. Although a number of doctors treated such cases as parasitic infections, Wyburn-Mason's work was never verified until recently. The latest research is now linking many cases of rheumatoid arthritis to intestinal parasites. Researchers at the New York University School of Medicine recently discovered that three-quarters of people with new-onset, untreated RA have *Prevotella copri* bacteria present in their intestinal tracts, plus reduced levels of several groups of beneficial microbes such as *Bacteroides*.[19]

Suspect this as the cause of your arthritis: if you have a mouth full of amalgam fillings (mercury has been shown to alter the gut's ecology) or elimination diets don't help you find the culprit.

Diagnose this: by getting your stools tested for parasites. Contact Biolab or Genova Diagnostics (*see page 95*).

Solve this: by taking a herbal formula, for several months (*see below*).

A herbal solution to parasites

If you've had a test for parasites and it comes back positive, here's the *What Doctors Don't Tell You* medical detective Harald Gaier's favourite formula for most gut bugs:

On weeks 1 and 3, take:

⇨ *Berberis vulgaris* (barberry) tincture (15ml three times/day)

⇨ Oregano oil (1 capsule a day), shown to inhibit parasites such as *Giardia*

⇨ *Artemisia absinthium* (wormwood) tincture (15ml three times/day)

⇨ Clove powder (one capsule a day)

On weeks 2 and 4, take:

⇨ *Hydrastis canadensis* (goldenseal) tincture (15ml three times/day)

⇨ Olive leaf extract (one capsule a day)

⇨ l-Glutamine (5g/day)

Berberis can attack all manner of gut bacteria, protozoans and yeasts,[20] as can *Artemisia*, and to these you might add a supplement of propolis, which works well against *Giardia*.[21] According to Essex-based medical herbalist Susan Koten, you should also consider seeing a herbalist to obtain a gallbladder flush made up of fringetree (*Chionanthus virginicus*), *Leptandra virginica* (Culver's root) and *Berberis vulgaris*, as the gallbladder is also often affected.

Candida albicans overgrowth

'When all you've got is a hammer, everything starts looking like a nail.' So said British nutritional pioneer Dr Stephen Davies about *Candida albicans* infection and the tendency of many doctors and alternative practitioners to diagnose anyone suffering from a collection of unexplained symptoms as victims of 'yeast syndrome'.

Some 25 years after Dr Orian Truss of Birmingham, Alabama, first theorized that overgrowth of the normally harmless *Candida* fungal yeast can wreak untold havoc in the gut, nutritional specialists such as UK naturopath Dr Harald Gaier now believe the situation is rather more complex. Candida may be only one of several culprits, and so-called 'candidiasis' sufferers may have several, quite distinct problems, including those listed in this book.

Suspect this as the cause of your arthritis: if your symptoms don't improve on an anti-inflamation diet (*see page 97*).

Diagnose this: by having a gut fermentation test. This measures whether you ferment ethyl alcohol in your gut after consuming glucose sugars, as often happens with yeast overgrowth. The test can distinguish yeast from simple bacterial overgrowth. (It can be done by Biolab: *see page 95.* In North America, Genova Diagnostics – again, *see page 95* – offers a candida antibody test, a simple saliva test that can confirm whether it's candida or not.)

Solve this: by killing candida with a natural antifungal, such as barberry (*Berberis*) tincture (15ml twice a day). Besides this, caprylic acid, goldenseal and a number of other traditional treatments have shown promise, including tea tree oil (*Melaleuca alternifolia*), oregano oil, proven to have potent anti-candida effects, and oil of cloves.[22]

Follow a low-carb diet and be sure to avoid sugars, yeast, alcohol and the usual allergy-related foods and, for a week or two, fruit. Check your nutritional status and take supplements if necessary. Integrative doctors find that their patients with candida are usually deficient in magnesium, zinc, vitamins A, B1 and B6, and omega-6 fatty acids. Take pancreatic enzymes (called 'proteases'), which also help to keep the small intestine free of parasites and aid digestion.[23] A lack of adequate digestive enzymes greatly increases the risk of intestinal infections, including chronic candida infections.

Add supplements of choline, betaine and methionine to clean up the workings of your liver, as chronic candida can lead to mild liver damage, at least in laboratory animals.[24] These liver enzymes boost your levels of two important antioxidants: S-adenosylmethionine[25] and glutathione.

Extract of milk thistle (*Silybum marianum*) at recommended dosages of between 70–210mg three times a day can stimulate the formation of new liver cells, and increase the production of glutathione and bile. It can also reduce liver injury.[26]

Where to get tested

The following laboratories carry out most of the tests recommended in this chapter, either in person or via post. Ideally, you will work with a qualified, experienced practitioner who will analyse which tests you need.

In the UK:

Biolab Medical Unit
The Stone House
9 Weymouth St
London W1N 3FF
020 7636 5959
www.biolab.co.uk

Genova Diagnostics Europe
Parkgate House
356 West Barnes Lane
New Malden
Surrey KT3 6NB
020 8336 7750
www.gdx.net/uk

In the USA:

Genova Diagnostics
63 Zillicoa Street
Suite A
Asheville, NC 28801-1074
800 522 4762
www.gdx.net

Chapter 7

THE ROLE OF DIET

As we've seen in the last section, dealing with arthritis is, to a great degree, about dealing with inflammation in your body. Most of the dietary, supplemental and lifestyle changes recommended in this book to prevent or heal arthritis start by food choices that heal inflammation.

Eat to heal

The anti-inflammation diet is fairly close to the already popular Mediterranean Diet, which consists primarily of fish, fruit, vegetables, cereals, beans and neutral fats. In those with rheumatoid arthritis, it's been associated with as much as a 56 per cent reduction in symptoms like joint swelling, tenderness and pain, and with better movement and vitality.[1] One reason may be that this largely plant-based diet is high in certain anti-inflammatory compounds, such as essential fatty acids and enzymes.

Before jumping in, however, and making radical dietary changes, bear in mind that the most effective approach is to introduce change gradually. If you quit toxic and inflammatory foods overnight, not only can your body go into a rapid detoxification reaction – temporarily bringing into your life detox symptoms such as headaches and joint pain and stiffness (some of the very things you're trying to avoid) – but also you probably won't last very long on the new programme anyway because the change will just seem too difficult. Avoid self-sabotage by taking at least a month to cut out fast foods and over-processed foods laden with bad fats, additives, sugars and wheat. Slowly replace processed foods with whole foods, fruits, vegetables and grains. And don't let the slogan 'whole grain' in breads and other supermarket products fool you since many so-called 'whole grain' breads are laden with sugar and many additives and artificial ingredients.

As you progress, take notes of your reactions. How do you feel? What do you crave? What symptoms are disappearing? After six weeks off all the hyper-inflammatory food, if you want to determine which foods in particular don't work for your body, you can try reintroducing them, one by one. Notice what reactions your body has (if any) to a food reintroduction. For example, does re-introducing milk in your tea bring on a big case of the snuffles, causing you to reach for the tissues again? If so, this is a big clue that your body is lactose-intolerant. Similar discoveries can be made by reintroducing potatoes and tomatoes and other nightshades. Do little aches and pains suddenly come back?

Mix it up. Try to eat different foods every day. This helps ensure you're getting all the vital nutrients your body needs, and helps you to stick to your new diet plan to keep your meals interesting. Eat several kinds of vegetables at one meal, and remember that most vegetables serve to increase the alkalinity of your body, which helps reduce inflammation. Make sure to get enough fibre in your diet by eating fruit, vegetables, whole grains, legumes and seeds – and don't forget to drink plenty of pure (filtered) water.

Foods to avoid

Avoid the following foods, which boost inflammation in your body:

⇨ Alcohol

⇨ All carbonated soft drinks and mixers, diet or otherwise

⇨ Artificial additives, including MSG, autolized yeast, hydrolyzed vegetable protein, parabens, glutamate, sodium caseinate and mineral oil

⇨ Aubergines

⇨ Breads, bagels, biscuits and the like

⇨ Confectionery/sweets

⇨ Cakes

⇨ Cereals (except oatmeal)

⇨ Coffee and black tea (switch to green or white)

⇨ Corn

⇨ Corn oil

⇨ Corn syrup

⇨ Crackers

⇨ Dairy products

⇨ Fried foods

⇨ Fruit juices (eat the whole fruit instead)

⇨ Flour (those containing gluten, such as wheat)

⇨ All gluten-containing grains

⇨ High-acid fruits

⇨ Mouldy foods

⇨ Noodles/pasta

⇨ Oils and foods made with omega-6 fatty acids, like sunflower oil: reduce these, and instead favour a higher intake of omega-3 fatty acids

⇨ Pizza

⇨ Red meats

⇨ Safflower oil

⇨ Soy products

⇨ Sugar (white and brown)

⇨ Tomatoes

⇨ Yeast

Not all flesh food needs to be avoided. Organic chicken, organic turkey, wild game, and wild-caught deep-sea fish, including salmon, tuna, herring and halibut (all sources of EPA, or eicosapentaenoic acid, and DHA, or docosahexaenoic acid), are healthy protein choices. Among red meats, only those high in a specific fatty acid (arachidonic acid) are believed to promote inflammation in the body.

When looking for a dairy substitute, experiment with dairy alternatives such as unsweetened almond milk, rice milk, hemp milk and coconut milk. Most people are at least somewhat lactose-intolerant and don't know it. If, having eliminated all dairy from your diet for six weeks, you want to experiment and see if your body can handle it, try reintroducing whole, raw (that is, unpasteurized) milk products from a reputable organic supplier.

If there is one dairy product more essential than others, it's butter, for the health-giving saturated fats. Homemade probiotic-rich kefirs and yogurts are great for gut health too, and incredibly easy to make. However, only dark chocolate, not milk chocolate, eaten in reasonable amounts and sweetened with honey or other non-inflammatory sweeteners, is non-inflammatory and good for you.

There's increasing evidence that a vegetarian or vegan diet can help to heal arthritis. Revealingly, researchers have found that a vegan, gluten-free diet can lead to up to a 10-fold increase in the rate of rheumatoid arthritis patients showing symptom improvement.[2]

Drinks to avoid

Besides avoiding certain foods, you also need to avoid a number of drinks that are pro-inflammatory. One of the greatest culprits is carbonated soft drinks.

After assessing the diets and lifestyles of 2,149 people with osteoarthritis in the knee joints, researchers discovered that carbonated drinks speed the progress of the disease, especially in men. Drinking just one sugary carbonated drink a day seems to quicken the disease and make the symptoms worse, particularly in men who aren't obese. Researchers from the Brigham and Women's Hospital and Tufts Medical Center in Boston, Massachusetts, and Brown University, Rhode Island, reported that the more carbonated drinks non-obese men had, the worse their symptoms became.[3]

Coffee drinkers may also face a higher risk of rheumatoid arthritis in later life, say Finnish researchers after studying nearly 26,000 individuals over 15 years. Those who drink four or more cups of coffee daily are twice as likely as occasional drinkers to test positive for arthritis. Anyone gulping down 11 or more cups a day was almost 15 times as likely to have high levels of rheumatoid factor circulating in their blood – a hallmark early sign of rheumatoid arthritis.[4]

Tap water

Making coffee or tea with tap water and even some bottled waters is a potential formula for arthritis too. Fluoride is added to municipal water supplies and even some bottled waters.

After studying 112 people with fluorosis, researchers have drawn up a list of symptoms of the early stages of fluorosis poisoning[5] that usually manifest before bone damage, including musculoskeletal problems such as:

⇨ Arthritis (cervical and lumbar spine)

⇨ Muscle pain

⇨ Pins and needles

⇨ Inability to control extremities

General symptoms of fluorosis include: coughing, excess mucus, breathing difficulties, mouth ulcers, bleeding gums, palpitations, vertigo, sleep problems, excessive thirst, excessive urination, joint pain, rash, memory loss, tinnitus (persistent ringing in the ears) and fatigue.

Foods to eat

Vegetables lead the list of anti-arthritis/anti-inflammatory foods to eat, especially dark leafy greens and brightly coloured veggies – Swiss chard, kale, spinach, rocket, beetroot, peppers (unless you are allergic to nightshades) and carrots – sweet potatoes (not white potatoes), yams, onions, parsnips, turnips, squashes (summer and winter), pumpkins and shitake mushrooms. Cruciferous vegetables such as broccoli and Brussels sprouts are particularly healing for arthritis conditions, as are asparagus, pak choi (bok choy in the USA), cauliflower, celery, cabbage and fennel. Kelp should be added to the list as well.

One vegetable in particular is an arthritis-fighting champion. Studies have found that eating a serving of broccoli every day could prevent and slow the spread of osteoarthritis. Sulphoraphane, a compound in the vegetable, slows the destruction of joint cartilage by blocking enzymes and interfering with the inflammatory processes associated with osteoarthritis. Sulphoraphane is also found in Brussels sprouts and cabbage.

Researchers from the University of East Anglia calculate that eating 100g (3.5oz) of broccoli, the equivalent to a handful, every day might prevent the disease or even slow its progress once it's been diagnosed.

After successfully demonstrating the positive effects of sulphoraphane in laboratory and animal trials,[6] researchers are now considering giving patients with osteoarthritis 'supercharged' broccoli – a specially grown variety that's a cross between standard broccoli and the wild broccoli found in Sicily,[7] in the hope that they'll see the disease slow and joints start to repair.

Besides vegetables, certain fruits help to put out your body's fire as well. Brightly coloured berries are the best for dealing with inflammation, and they also contain lots of antioxidants and phytonutrients. Blueberries are especially potent, but red and black raspberries, strawberries, blackberries, salmonberries, grapes and currants are good choices as well. Pineapple, kiwi, papaya and apricots (which contain the anti-inflammatory phytochemical known as quercetin) are all specific inflammation-fighters. If you're not sensitive to citric acid, lemons and limes are good choices, as are oranges and grapefruit. Avocados are incredibly delicious fruits that are anti-inflammatory, contain healthy fats and are one of the healthiest foods on the planet. Cantaloupe melons are filled with phytonutrients, antioxidants, and vitamins A and C, all highly anti-inflammatory. New evidence supports the view that phytonutrients, antioxidants and various vitamins can help to protect you from developing arthritis.[8]

As for grains, opt for gluten-free grains like millet, quinoa, whole rice (black, brown or red) and wild rice, amaranth and buckwheat. Beans and legumes, such as black beans, chickpeas (garbanzo beans), kidney beans, lima beans, lentils and peas, are a hearty substitute for refined gluten products and are also good sources of protein and fibre.

The best protein choices include eggs, organic chicken, organic turkey, wild game, and wild-caught deep-sea fish, including salmon, tuna, herring and halibut. Oysters and prawns, in moderation, are also fine.

Non-inflammatory sweeteners include honey, brown rice syrup, coconut syrup, maple syrup, molasses, Xylitol and Stevia. Use healthy oils such as coconut oil, olive oil, avocado oil, organic butter/ghee and lard. Omega-3-rich oils cold-pressed from algae, fish and seeds (chia, flax, hemp, pumpkin and so on) are also an essential part of a healthy inflammation-free diet. Healthy nuts and seeds include almonds, cashews, walnuts, flax and chia.

The most anti-inflammatory spices include turmeric, curcumin, cinnamon and ginger.

Foods for gout

It's important for people with gout to follow a low-acid diet, avoiding foods that are rich in purines, the chemicals the body converts to uric acid, which lead to the formation of crystals in joints, resulting in pain and inflammation.

In one study, substitution of a purine-free formula diet over a period of days reduced the blood-uric-acid levels of healthy men from an average of 5.0mg/dl to 3.0mg/dl.9 This can prevent attacks of gout from recurring. Drinking six to eight glasses of water a day also helps, as this will dilute uric-acid levels in the blood.

A traditional remedy for gout is consuming one half to one pound (225–250g) of sweet cherries a day. While the US Food and Drug Administration (FDA) is unconvinced of the health benefits of this fruit, a recent small study has supported cherries' reputed anti-gout action.[10] Celery juice (or celery seed) is another folk remedy for gout that's apparently widely used in Australia.

The power of fasting

Carrying out intermittent fasting is a final change to your diet that may offer a powerful way to mitigate arthritis symptoms.

Studies at the University of Oslo have found benefits from a short fast followed by dietary changes in alleviating symptoms of rheumatoid arthritis.[11] In one two-year study, improvement was noted in patients with rheumatoid arthritis after fasting followed by an individually adjusted vegetarian diet for a year. Follow-up a year later showed that the benefit remained for a subset of those who had stuck to the vegetarian diet.[12]

Fasting for just two days can kick-start the immune system – and might reverse autoimmune conditions such as arthritis. Going without food for two to four days kills older and damaged immune cells while generating new ones. At the beginning of a fast, white blood cells are killed off before a 'regenerative switch' is flipped, which alters the signalling pathways of stem cells responsible for the generation of blood and immune-system cells.

Other extensive changes in the diet after a fast have also been investigated, particularly cutting out meat. A review of four studies looking at the effect of brief fasting followed by at least three months on a vegetarian diet showed 'a statistically and clinically significant beneficial long-term effect'.[13]

Fasting, followed by a vegan diet, may also have a positive effect on gut flora, that population of microbes in your gut. One Norwegian study followed patients with rheumatoid arthritis who were asked to fast for seven to 10 days, then follow a vegan diet for three and a half months and finally to adhere to a lacto-vegetarian diet for a further nine months. The Norwegian researchers discovered improvements in the patients, which couldn't be explained by any changes in immune-system activity. However, 'the faecal flora differed significantly between samples collected at time points at which there was substantial clinical improvement,' noted the researchers, suggesting that the state of your microbiome plays a major role in exacerbating or healing arthritis.[14]

Fasting could be an important strategy for anyone with an immune deficiency, including autoimmune disorders such as arthritis, say researchers from the University of Southern California's School of Gerontology. The researchers were astonished by the health benefits of fasting, which they measured with two-, three- and four-day fasts. They suspect that fasting might benefit all of the body's organs, and not just the immune system.[15]

You can fast by consuming only juices (made up of allowed fruits or vegetables) or simply water. If you choose to do a fast, don't just go cold turkey. Make sure to slowly wind down your consumption of food to light proteins, vegetables and whole grains before entering the fast, and do the same in reverse once you break the fast. If you intend to fast for more than three or four days, be sure to work with an experienced, qualified professional, who can monitor your progress.

Arthritis and the great fat debate

Back in the 1980s, when Dr Collin H. Dong developed a simple diet similar to that followed by ancestral Chinese peasants, his 'caveman diet' excluded meat, fruit, dairy products, vinegar and other acids, peppers, hot spices, chocolate, dry-roasted nuts, alcohol and soft drinks, and was high in fish and fish oils.

In her book *Diet for Life*[16], a cookbook for arthritis sufferers, Mary Laver, a patient of Dr Collin H. Dong's, based in England, describes how she recovered from arthritis after faithfully following this regime. Laver says the diet takes from three to six weeks to work. When the diet is working, she tells us, there's a foul taste in the mouth caused by the elimination of toxins from the system. Laver claims that the diet didn't cure her arthritis (her blood tests remain positive today), but it ended her symptoms of stiffness and pain.

||||||||||||||||||||||||||||||||||||||||||||

Chapter 8

HEALING WITH ESSENTIAL FATTY ACIDS

Before the millennium, the US National Institutes of Health (NIH) recommended an upper limit of 6.7g/day of omega-6 fatty acids – equivalent to around 3 per cent of the calories in the average person's diet. In January 2009, the American Heart Association (AHA) and other medical professionals nearly tripled that recommended level, exhorting Americans to take at least '5 per cent to 10 per cent of their calories from omega-6 fatty acids'.[1]

Depending on the level of physical activity, age and gender, this works out as 12–22g/day.

But several decades of research into this relatively new field tell a more sober and complicated story. Far from aiding health, such high levels of one type of fat over the other can create health problems as serious as those caused by the excess consumption of the 'fake fats' – that is, trans fatty acids.

Researchers now blame the imbalance between omega-3 and -6 fatty acids for many cases of heart disease, high blood pressure, diabetes and obesity, and other inflammatory diseases such as arthritis. Excessive omega-6 supplementation may even be a major cause of depression and bipolar disorder. Consequently, one of the cornerstones of any healing diet for arthritis is making sure you are consuming the right ratio of essential fats.

The basic omega fats

Up until the turn of the 21st century, doctors believed that omega-6 was the most important essential fatty acid (EFA) because of its supposedly anti-inflammatory, blood-thinning and vascular-dilating properties.

In 1993, the World Health Organization (WHO) sponsored an international team of experts, who concluded that 'desirable intakes of linoleic acid should provide between 4 and 10 per cent of energy' and 'the ratio of linoleic to alpha-linolenic acids in the diet should be between 5:1 and 10:1 (omega-6 to omega-3)'.

Consequently, for several decades, Westerners – Americans in particular – have been told to use omega-6 fats whenever possible in place of saturated fats. This has resulted in an average ratio for Americans these days of 20:1 and, in some cases, even 50:1, of omega-6 to omega-3 fats. And this ratio is increasing in favour of omega-6s, as Americans now eschew eating seafish, the richest source of omega-3 EFAs, because of the increased likelihood of contamination and pollution.

More heart disease

New evidence has emerged showing that, far from being protective, a high omega-6 consumption is linked to a massive increase in inflammatory diseases such as heart disease and arthritis. In the famous Lyon Diet Heart Study, French heart patients were given either the AHA's polyunsaturated fats-rich 'heart diet' or the Mediterranean diet, the latter replacing polyunsaturated fats with olive oil, which is rich in oleic acid, an omega-9 monosaturated fat. Those eating the Mediterranean diet had an approximately 45 per cent reduction in deaths from any cause, including heart disease and cancer.[2]

The ongoing Massachusetts-based Framingham Heart Study found that those at risk of heart disease weren't protected by high omega-6 intakes. In fact, their atherosclerosis became worse.[3] It's now known that omega-6 fats can cause those with an inherited atherosclerotic tendency to blossom into disease: people with a particular genotype (5-lipoxy-genase, or LOX) develop hardened arteries with high levels of omega-6, whereas omega-3 is protective.[4]

High intakes of omega-6 fats are also related to an increase in heart disease. A Finnish study found a link between high omega-6 consumption and increased oxidation of low-density lipoproteins. (LDL; the bad, atherogenic type of cholesterol).[5]

Dangers of excessive omega-6 fatty acids

Besides heart disease, no less than three large-scale studies have shown that excessive levels of omega-6 fatty acids – such as currently recommended by the AHA – have been linked to breast cancer.

In a recent Swedish study, high omega-6 intakes – more than 17.4g/day – doubled the incidence of breast cancer among those women who were genetically susceptible.[6]

This evidence suggests that, far from reducing inflammation, excess omega-6s bring about chronic inflammation in the body, leading to a plethora of disease states, including arthritis.

Omega-3 protection

In stark contrast, the omega-3 fats have an impressive amount of research to support their protective effects. Fish oils have been shown to decrease the incidence of acute coronary events such as heart attack and sudden cardiac death,[7] and to prevent depression and cancer. They have also proved helpful in combatting a host of diseases, including Crohn's disease, ulcerative colitis and rheumatoid arthritis.[8] Fish oils have been shown to improve joint function in patients with rheumatoid arthritis.[9]

Wrong ratio

Researchers have now begun to question whether omega-6s are truly necessary for human health. New evidence suggests that the initial research on omega-6 overestimated the amount needed by the body.[10]

In fact, most scientists now maintain that the problem isn't omega-6 fatty acids per se, since these are necessary for human health, so much as a massive overdose of them, which virtually eliminates the body's store of omega-3. It's known that the two fats compete with each other for enzymes to be converted into useful products in the body.

This is a point of particular concern, as the average daily British or American diet is already low on omega-3 – amounting to only one eighth of the 650mg/day of EPA and DHA recommended by the US NIH.

The diet of our ancestors was rich in omega-3, with a typical ratio of omega-6s to omega-3s of 1:1, compared with the average ratio in the USA and UK now of 1:15 to 1:16. A ratio of 4:1, for example, has been associated with a 70 per cent decrease in total mortality.

Nevertheless, there may not be a one-size-fits-all ratio for everyone. Different diseases respond to different ratios of omega-6 to omega-3 fats, and the optimal ratio appears to depend on how ill you are – the more severe the disease, the lower the ratio (closer to 1:1) required.

Patients with asthma found that a ratio of 5:1 was beneficial (while a ratio of 10:1 was shown to worsen their condition). For those with rheumatoid arthritis, a 5:1 ratio had no effect, whereas a ratio of 2–3:1 suppressed inflammation. An even lower ratio was able to reduce the spread of cancer.

Here are some EFA guidelines to help you keep inflammation at bay:

Attempt a ratio of 1:1 omega-6 to omega-3: This is usually optimum, but the amount you take should depend on your state of health.

Take your body weight into account: If you're ill, nutritionists recommend 300mg of EPA and DHA for every 4.5kg (10lb) of body weight. This equates to 1tbsp of your average cod liver oil, or 10 capsules, for a 59kg (130lb) person.

Use olive oil: This is the healthy option, instead of polyunsaturated fatty acids (PUFAs), for cooking.

Take omega-3s with vitamin E: As EFAs are fragile and easily oxidized, leading to harmful free radicals, always take them in a supplement using naturally derived vitamin E, which mops up free radicals.

Remember your vitamins B and C: Since EFAs require other essential nutrients to be adequately utilized in the body, make sure that you're taking adequate amounts of vitamins B and C, as well as magnesium, calcium and zinc.

Choose the right fish oil: Ensure that your brand of fish oil is free of mercury and polycarbon biphenols (PCBs) – pollutants from industry, which make their way into seafood. This will require some detective work, such as contacting the manufacturer and checking out independent reports of the product.

Flaxseed vs fish oil

If you're vegetarian, you can take flaxseed or walnut oil as your source of omega-3, but be aware that both oils contain the precursor alpha-linolenic acid (ALA), which needs to be converted to EPA and DHA for optimal benefit. This conversion process isn't particularly efficient, and it gets worse with age,[11] especially if you also have raised insulin levels, as these will inhibit delta-6-desaturase, the enzyme necessary to convert ALA to EPA and DHA.

A sensible guideline for dietary fats

Hopefully, it should be obvious that most people could do with a major rethink of their daily dietary fat intake. If you're worried about developing arthritis or are already dealing with the disease, all the more reason to take heed. For some people this will mean cutting back, while for others it will mean completely reorganizing their diets to eat more or different types of fats. Here are a few pointers that should help:

Trans fatty acids are the only truly bad fats: Only trans fatty acids – the 'fake', man-made hydrogenated oils, as distinct from the saturates that occur naturally in animal flesh, nuts and dairy products – have been consistently proven to cause atherosclerosis and other health issues that, like arthritis, are linked to inflammation.[12]

Best fats for cooking and general use are: high-quality, extra virgin olive oil for low-heat cooking; and coconut, palm or avocado oil and organic butter or ghee for all high-heat cooking.

Omega-3 is essential: Avoid drowning in omega-6 and worsening your omega-6 (linoleic acid, LA) to omega-3 (alpha-linolenic acid, ALA) ratio. Cut down or eliminate vegetable oils, spreads and shortenings that contain sunflower, corn, soy, safflower or canola oils. Hemp seeds contain a healthy proportion of omega-6 to omega-3 fatty acids, with a ratio ranging from 2:1 to 3:1. Krill oil has the best omega-6 to -3 ratio.

Omega-3 supplementation can benefit a range of inflammatory conditions, including rheumatoid arthritis. Although initially sceptical about fish oils, rheumatologists have taken the claims seriously enough to do proper clinical trials. After pooling the data, their unequivocal conclusion was that taking fish-oil supplements for three months 'significantly' reduced joint pain and stiffness in rheumatoid arthritis patients – with no side effects.[13] Taking these supplements improved joint function and lowered the need for

NSAID use.[14] But even regular consumption of EFAs in grilled or baked fish seems to reduce the risk of rheumatoid arthritis in women. The key beneficial ingredient in fish, whether in supplement or food form, is believed to be the omega-3 fatty acids.[15]

In another trial, krill oil was tested against a placebo for its anti-inflammatory effects. Ninety patients with cardiovascular disease, rheumatoid arthritis or osteoarthritis, along with high levels of C-reactive protein, or CRP, a marker of systemic inflammation, were given either 300mg/day of krill oil or a placebo for 30 days. By day seven, krill oil had significantly reduced CRP (by 19 per cent) compared to the placebo. By day 30, krill oil had further reduced CRP by 30 per cent. The researchers also reported reduced arthritic symptoms in the krill oil group, including less pain, stiffness and functional impairment.[16]

Besides supplements, look to dietary sources of omega-3. In fact, if you are an avid fish eater, it may be possible to get all of the omega-3 fatty acids from your diet. Try eating two portions a week of oil-rich fish (salmon, mackerel, herring, sardines, tuna and black cod, or sablefish). This will provide around 2–3g of very-long-chain fatty acids – the amount found in three or four 1000mg fish-oil capsules. Organically reared, grass-fed animals, eggs from grain-fed chickens and wild (not farmed) fish and game will also provide useful amounts of this and other naturally occurring fats.

Some additional guidelines on oils

Variety is the key: Your best health insurance policy is to get dietary fats from a wide variety of sources.

Organic is best: Many industrial pollutants are lipophilic – meaning that they are attracted to fat. This means that animal fats, dairy products, seed and fish oils may be substantially polluted with toxins such as pesticides, dioxins, polychlorinated biphenyls (PCBs) and xenoestrogens. To get the best out of whatever fats you eat, choose organic wherever possible.

Sensible supplementing makes sense: If you're worried about high-dose supplementing, a good compromise is to take half your requirements from food and half from supplements.

Take vitamin E: Fish-oil supplementation has been said to lower blood concentrations of vitamin E and other fat-soluble nutrients such as retinol and beta-carotene, so it's prudent to add an extra 200mg of vitamin E to your regime.

Go Mediterranean: There's ample evidence that olive oil, too, relieves pain and may also reduce the risk of developing rheumatoid arthritis if consumed regularly.[17]

The 'designer' fats

Besides fish oils, consider adding a few other oils to your diet:

CMO, or **Cetyl myristoleate**: Widely touted on the Internet as a 'designer fat' or 'super lubricant,' CMO is basically an oil. An essential fatty acid found in fish oils and butter, CMO is a component of the unsaturated fatty acid cis-9-tetra-decanoic acid (myristoleic acid). It's present in sebum, the oily secretion of our skin.

CMO was first discovered by Dr Harry W. Diehl, a scientist at the US National Institutes of Health, who'd embarked on a crusade to find a cure for arthritis. He's best known for synthesizing a type of sugar used to prepare the oral polio vaccine.

After years of what he termed 'chemical sleuthing', Dr Diehl isolated CMO. This substance, which had never been identified before, is abundant in the blood of mice and was the factor, he postulated, that protected them against arthritis.

Dr Len Sands, former Director of the International Immunological Center of the San Diego Clinic, conducted a series of CMO trials at the clinic in the 1990s and created an oral version of CMO. One basic cause for concern about the CMO craze is that no one has any real idea of how it works. Clearly, more research is needed into this potentially useful substance.

Cetylated fatty acids: These, abbreviated as CFAs, are another of the latest natural approaches for joint health and osteoarthritis. Several studies have been done on a product called Celadrin, a blend of 70 per cent CFAs to 30 per cent olive oil. In a study on its oral application, 64 patients with chronic knee osteoarthritis took either Celadrin (350mg, plus 50mg of soy lecithin and 75mg of fish oil) or a placebo. At the end of the study (68 days), those taking Celadrin improved their knee range of motion and overall joint functioning significantly in comparison to those in the placebo group, leading the authors to conclude that 'CFA may be an alternative to the use of non-steroidal anti-inflammatory drugs' for the treatment of osteoarthritis.'[18]

Researchers from the Human Performance Laboratory at the University of Connecticut conducted studies on how fast and long-lasting a topical cream version of Celadrin worked with patients (mean age: 65 years) suffering from knee osteoarthritis.

Tests included timing patients getting up from a sitting position, climbing stairs and other measures of knee mobility. Celadrin proved superior to the placebo and had fast-acting effects.[19]

Other lab studies found Celadrin in topical form to be effective for relieving the pain of osteoarthritis, as well as improving postural stability, weight distribution while standing,[20] and improved function in patients with osteoarthritis of the elbow and wrist.[21]

Emu oil: Emu oil is a product rendered from the fat of the flightless emu bird native to Australia that Australian aborigines have used to heal wounds, reduce pain and relieve muscle problems for centuries. It's a combination of oleic acid (an omega-9 monounsaturated fatty acid), polyunsaturated fatty acids linoleic acid (omega-6 fat) and linolenic acid (omega-3 fat), as well as the saturated fatty acids palmitic acid and stearic acid. Few scientific tests have been conducted on emu oil, and most of those have been done on animals.

Australian researchers tested five different emu-oil preparations on rats with epolyarthritis (arthritis involving multiple joints). Four out of the five oils effectively reduced arthritic symptoms in a manner comparable to taking the anti-inflammatory drug ibuprofen.[22]

||||||||||||||||||||||||||||||||||||||||||||||||

Part III

ALTERNATIVE TREATMENTS FOR ARTHRITIS

Chapter 9

THE BEST ALTERNATIVES

Given the persistent problems with conventional treatments, it's little wonder that many arthritis sufferers have looked to alternative medicine for help. One recent study carried out at the University of St Joseph in Beirut, Lebanon, found that 23 per cent of a sampling of patients used alternative treatments for their arthritis, 64 per cent of whom believed that the complementary alternative therapy was beneficial.[1]

While 'official' organizations such as the Arthritis Foundation pooh-pooh all but the most widely used conventional treatments, the sheer pandemic proportions of arthritis and the wide variety of different kinds of arthritis make it clear that considering other solutions is necessary and desirable.

In spite of all this, the official line is that there are no other 'cures' for arthritis and that anything other than the accepted pathway is just quackery. The Arthritis Foundation believes that most of the people who have sought an alternative have failed to find relief. Their attitude wrongly assumes that copper bracelets and motor oil can happily be lumped in together with acupuncture, yoga and herbs; and that conventional medicine is some sort of haven for sufferers.

These views fail to acknowledge that perhaps 90 per cent of sufferers feel, in some way, let down by the conventional approach and its myriad unpleasant side effects. It also ignores those studies that show that arthritis sufferers can find relief from pain, stiffness and inflammation through a variety of alternative methods, either singly or in combination.

What follows is not a definitive guide to the alternative therapies available, but coverage of those that have a reasonable, scientific body of evidence to suggest that they may either reduce the pain and severity of arthritis or actually cause the debilitating disease to disappear altogether.

Acupuncture

Acupuncture is an ancient traditional Chinese medical (TCM) technique based on the concept that all life forms are supported by subtle energy known as *chi* or *qi*. In TCM, blockages or excesses of energy at certain points and organs of the body are understood to result in illness. The blocks and excesses of chi are balanced by inserting incredibly thin needles placed into acupuncture points – specific places along the body's meridians (energy lines).

Because of its known analgesic effects, acupuncture is widely used for arthritis. Proper clinical trials are thin on the ground, but most research studies that have been carried out on acupuncture treatments for arthritis are generally positive.

Dramatic results were reported by Scandinavian doctors on patients whose osteoarthritis was so severe that they were scheduled for surgery. Astonishingly for such advanced cases, monthly acupuncture was found to relieve as much as 80 per cent of the pain.[2]

Similar benefits were found by doctors at the Princess Margaret Hospital in Swindon, Wiltshire, in the UK, who studied a group of patients with advanced osteoarthritis of the hip. Six half-hour acupuncture sessions eased their pain and improved their mobility for up to eight weeks after treatment.[3]

One technique sometimes used by acupuncturists who specialize in arthritis is to put bee venom on the ends of their needles before inserting them. Experiments on arthritic laboratory rats have confirmed the value of this novel approach.[4]

Bee venom acupuncture, which delivers compounds isolated from bee venom directly into an acupoint, can reduce the pain and swelling associated with arthritis.[5] In patients with osteoarthritis of the knee, four weeks of bee venom acupuncture has been demonstrated to be more effective at relieving pain than traditional needle acupuncture.[6]

Strange as it may seem, there's a logical reason for the bee venom approach to work – at least from the perspective of homeopathic treatment, which uses the 'law of similarities' to accomplish healing of a wide variety of diseases. According to homeopathy, things found in nature – not only plants and herbs, but even toxins from bees and other insects and animals or substances that create reactions in the body – can be used to treat and cure the same kinds of reactions they cause.

A bee sting causes inflammation, heat, swelling and pain. Accordingly, the 'law of similarities' dictates that bee venom can be used to treat any condition (such as arthritis) that causes the same kinds of symptoms.

More recent studies suggest that acupuncture might also help those who have shoulder pain, headaches, temporomandibular joint (TMJ) dysfunction, fibromyalgia, osteoarthritis of the knee, tennis/golfer's elbow and other painful conditions involving inflamed joints.[7]

Acupuncture for knee arthritis

Acupuncture can relieve the pain of knee osteoarthritis so effectively that surgery isn't needed. During one study, patients of acupuncture said they weren't feeling any pain as much as two years after acupuncture treatments for their knee arthritis – whereas, by then, one in seven of those who underwent conventional surgery complained of suffering severe pain.

One group of 90 sufferers, with an average age of 71 years, was treated with acupuncture. In each case, the arthritis was so severe that it warranted surgery. Instead, they were given acupuncture once a week for a month and then once every six weeks. All of the patients reported a dramatic reduction in pain and stiffness, and an improvement in mobility – in fact, the improvements were so dramatic that none of them needed surgery. Of this group of people, 31 were still having regular acupuncture sessions two years later.[8]

Researchers at the Sloan-Kettering Cancer Center in New York collated 29 different randomized controlled trial (RCT) studies involving 17,922 patients who were given either acupuncture or 'sham' acupuncture (whereby the needles either weren't inserted properly or were put in 'wrong' places on the body).

The patients given real acupuncture reported a far greater reduction in their pain than those given sham acupuncture, demonstrating that it was the actual therapy – and not the placebo effect – that was working.[9]

The huge volume of research that's been carried out convinced the Sloan-Kettering researchers that acupuncture eases chronic pain and that its effects are real and have nothing to do with the placebo effect. Presently, they recommend the inclusion of acupuncture in the range of pain-control options offered to patients.

Finally, in one study it was found that people who underwent one month of acupuncture treatment had a greater reduction of uric acid and other markers for gout than did a control group. The researchers concluded that acupuncture may also help prevent kidney damage from gout.[10]

Homeopathy

Research has shown that individually prescribed homeopathic remedies can help with arthritis, and some may enhance the effect of conventional treatments.[11]

A homeopathic approach to arthritis is holistic, which means that it doesn't just treat arthritis symptoms, but treats the whole person and the underlying causes of the condition, including physical, emotional and social conditions that might be contributing to susceptibility and illness.

Homeopathy also meticulously examines the problem itself and how it shows up. A homeopathic doctor doesn't just treat pain or swelling, but will look closer at the *kind* of pain. Is it stabbing, throbbing, dull, chronic, intermittent? Does it improve with exercise? Or does it worsen? Is there sleep disturbance accompanying the pain? Restlessness? Exhaustion accompanying the symptoms? Where's the pain located? How long has it been a problem? Does the pain move? Is there a pattern? Do foods seem to trigger symptoms?

Homeopathic prescriptions are all natural and highly individualized for each person's condition and symptom set. For individualized treatment you should, of course, consult a qualified homeopathic doctor in person. However, there are some important general remedies that are often recommended for treatment of arthritis. These include:

⇨ **Benzoic acid:** Used to treat gout-like conditions and pain from deposits of uric acid.

⇨ **Bryonia Alba:** Suitable for pain with inflammation made worse by movement, and eased by pressure and rest.

⇨ **Calc Carb:** Often prescribed for arthritic knees, especially in people who are overweight who complain of the condition being worse when they are cold.

⇨ **Colchicum:** For arthritis pain that's made worse by exercise, or even mental effort, and made better by warmth and rest.

⇨ **Guaiacum:** A remedy given for gout and joint abscesses when the pain is eased by cold.

⇨ **Hypericum:** Highly effective in reducing nerve pain from rheumatoid arthritis.

⇨ **Ledum pal:** Often used for gout and rheumatism and symptoms made better by application of ice or cold packs.

⇨ **Rhus tox:** Used in situations where initial movement is painful and made better by continuous motion.

⇨ **Paloondo:** A plant found in Mexico and southern California. Once used by the Aztecs for rheumatoid-arthritic conditions, it has been found useful for RA in homeopathic potencies.

Homeopathy for gout

For natural pain relief of gout, try the following homeopathic remedies:

⇨ **Aconite:** For sudden burning pain and attacks that come after a shock or injury.

⇨ **Belladonna:** For intense, throbbing pain.

⇨ **Bryonia:** For pain that's made worse by motion, but gets better with pressure and heat.

⇨ **Clochicum:** Especially good if there's nausea associated with the attacks.

⇨ **Ledum:** For joints that are mottled, purple and swollen. The usual dose of Ledum is three to five pellets of a 12X to 30C remedy, taken every one to four hours until the symptoms improve.[12]

Electromagnetism therapies

A century ago, electromagnetic fields were used extensively in medicine, but they were phased out with the rise of the drug-based approach to disease. In the last 20 years, however, they've begun a tentative comeback. To date, their major medical application has been in orthopaedics, where they've been used to help healing in bone fractures: applying magnetic fields can speed up the natural bone-healing process.

This discovery has sparked off a limited amount of research, with spin-offs for arthritis. In the laboratory, electromagnetic fields have been shown to stimulate the growth of both bone and cartilage.[13]

In hospital, the fact that patients can't tell whether an electromagnetic field generator is switched on or off makes the therapy ideal for blind controlled trials. One recent study looked at 176 people with osteoarthritis of the knee. An EM field generator was placed around the knee and switched on for half the patients, but left off for the other half. The treatment consisted of eight 48-minute EM sessions over two weeks. The results were very clear-cut: 46 per cent of the patients on the real treatment found their pain levels were reduced, compared to eight per cent on the sham procedure.[14]

Although the evidence is still relatively sparse, a 2013 review of the available data confirmed that EM therapy 'may provide moderate benefit for osteoarthritis sufferers in terms of pain relief'.[15]

The US National Center for Complementary and Alternative Medicine (NCCAM) identifies two types of energy medicine: 1) bioelectromagnetic-based therapies that use electromagnetic fields (EMFs) such as pulsed fields, magnetic fields and alternating/direct current fields, and 2) biofield therapies directed towards the energy fields that surround the entire body (also known as the aura).[16]

One other technique that falls into the EMF category is transcutaneous electrical nerve stimulation, or TENS, a practice whereby a therapist places electrodes on or near the painful areas and then runs a low-voltage electrical current between them. According to advocates, stimulating the nerves closes a 'gate' mechanism in the spinal cord, thus helping to eliminate the sensation of pain. Another theory is that nerve stimulation induces the body to produce the natural painkillers known as endorphins.

Numerous studies have shown that TENS works for a range of chronic pain conditions – from musculoskeletal pain, such as back and neck pain, to the persistent pain that often follows surgery.[17]

Of the other bioelectromagnetic-based therapies that are currently available, pulsed electromagnetic field (PEMF) generators and cranial electrotherapy stimulation (CES) hold particular promise for patients who suffer from chronic pain.

PEMF generators – which include low-power, wearable devices designed for virtually continuous use as well as high-power machines meant to be used several times a day – are able to help osteoarthritis sufferers.[18]

CES, which delivers a low-level electrical current through electrodes attached to the skin surface (usually on the ears), has proved to be better than a sham procedure for treating fibromyalgia pain as well as the pain associated with spinal cord injury.[19]

Precisely how these two electrical treatments work is still not fully understood. PEMF generators appear to increase blood flow to the areas exposed to the EMFs, whereas CES is thought to bring about changes in certain chemicals of the brain, including serotonin and norepinephrine.

Both mechanisms appear to have a positive effect on pain.[20]

Energy medicine

Other energetic approaches for arthritis pain include the ancient Chinese practice of qigong (Chi Gong), as well as Reiki and Therapeutic Touch. By combining slow, deliberate movements, meditation and regulated breathing, gigong enhances the flow of qi in the body with the specific goal of producing health and longevity.

The evidence for qigong is the most encouraging, with one study demonstrating that 91 per cent of patients with complex pain syndrome reporting pain relief compared to 36 per cent of patients given a sham treatment.[21]

A review of clinical trials showed that qigong had 'significant effects' compared to conventional care, in alleviating pain.[22]

Plant substances and extracts

The following botanically derived treatments are noteworthy:

Bromelain

Pineapple (*Ananas comosus*) has been used for centuries in Central and South America to treat indigestion and reduce inflammation.

Today, its extract bromelain is showing promise for a range of conditions, including arthritis.[23]

A mixture of proteolytic enzymes (enzymes that digest protein), bromelain may work better than most NSAIDs for reducing pain and improving function. As well as being a popular aid to digestion, bromelain appears to be a powerful anti-inflammatory, analgesic, antimicrobial and immune-system-boosting agent, which makes it a useful supplement for a variety of health conditions.

In a double-blind randomized study of 90 osteoarthritis patients, a supplement containing bromelain (90mg), along with the enzyme trypsin (48mg) and the flavonoid rutin (100mg), was compared with the non-steroidal anti-inflammatory drug (NSAID) diclofenac (50mg). After six weeks, the results showed that the enzyme supplement was just as effective as diclofenac for improving pain, joint stiffness and physical function – and the supplement was also better tolerated.[24]

Other evidence suggests that bromelain may be useful for rheumatoid arthritis too. In a small, uncontrolled study, bromelain was given to 29 patients with arthritic joint swelling (25 of whom had rheumatoid arthritis), for a period of three to 13 months. Added to the patients' steroid therapy in one study, bromelain resulted in a significant-to-complete reduction in soft tissue swelling in 21 of the patients.[25]

Bromelain has shown beneficial effects in doses as small as 160mg/day. However, it's thought that, for most conditions, the best results are seen with larger doses of 750–1,000mg/day – usually in four divided doses.[26] The German Commission E, a scientific advisory board for the German equivalent of the US

Food and Drug Administration, recommends 80–320mg two or three times a day (for adults), but other research recommends up to 2,000mg several times a day. For specific conditions, higher doses may be prescribed (but consult a qualified practitioner for a personal recommendation).

Suggested daily dosage: take 80–2,000mg/day in two divided doses

Black cumin

The botanical name for black cumin is *Nigella sativa*. Constituents in the oil and seeds – in particular, thymoquinine (TQ) – have shown potent anti-inflammatory effects in the laboratory.[27] In another study, 40 women with RA were given a placebo for a month, and then 500mg of *Nigella sativa* oil capsules twice a day and again a month's worth of a placebo. Disease activity, number of swollen joints and morning stiffness all improved, often markedly, during the time when *Nigella sativa* was given.[28]

Suggested daily dosage: 1 tsp of black cumin seed oil with meals

Curcumin

This yellow pigment, a natural phenolic compound derived from the turmeric plant (*Curcuma longa*), has long been used to treat joint inflammation in Ayurvedic medicine, the traditional system of medicine in India, because of its ability to halt cartilage destruction and reduce inflammation.[29] Overall, curcumin has been shown in over 50 clinical studies to have potent anti-inflammatory properties.

In one study of 21 patients with mild-to-moderate knee osteoarthritis, subjects were given either curcumin (1,500mg/day in three divided doses) or a matched placebo for six weeks. Those patients given the curcumin experienced significant improvements in pain and physical mobility compared to those patients given a placebo, with no major side effects.

Suggested daily dosage: 400–800mg

Ginger

This traditional herbal remedy, known scientifically as *Zingiber officinale*, has properties similar to those of non-steroidal anti-inflammatory drugs (NSAIDs), including the ability to interfere with the pathway that leads to chronic inflammation.[30]

Suggested daily dosage: 2–4g of fresh ginger juice, extract or tea

You can also rub ginger oil directly onto a painful joint, or make a warm poultice or compress of fresh ginger root and apply it to any painful areas.

Meta050

In an eight-week trial, this standardized combination of reduced iso-alpha-acids from hops, rosemary extract and oleanolic acid significantly relieved pain (by 40–50 per cent) in patients with rheumatoid arthritis, osteoarthritis and fibromyalgia.[31]

Suggested daily dosage: As in the trial, 440mg of Meta050 three times a day for four weeks, followed by 880mg twice a day for a further four weeks

Pycnogenol

An extract of French maritime pine bark, Pycnogenol reduced the pain and stiffness of mild osteoarthritis in one study. Those taking Pycnogenol were able to reduce their use of painkillers and carry out more of their everyday activities.[32]

Suggested daily dosage: as directed on product packaging or by a practitioner

Rosehip powder

Rosehip powder, derived from the fruit of the rose flower, has been shown to reduce symptoms of knee and hip osteoarthritis, including pain, stiffness, diability, global severity of symptoms and the need for 'rescue medicine'.[33]

Other herbal remedies that have shown promise in treating forms of arthritis include devil's claw, willow bark, Phytodolor (a fixed formulation containing alcoholic extracts of *Populus tremula*, *Fraxinus excelsior* and *Solidago virgaurea*), and capsaicin.[34]

A herbal formula based on *Boswellia* has been tested in osteoarthritis patients in several double-blind trials, with highly significant effects on pain and joint mobility.[35] The most recent study showed that patients including the herb formulation in addition to 'standard medical treatment' (that is, drugs) over 12 weeks were able significantly to extend their walking distance on a treadmill and also reduce their needs for drugs and medical attention.[36]

Devil's claw

Although the scientific evidence is mixed about the African plant *Harpagophytum procumbens* or *H. radix*, whose root is used for healing, one study in a review including five randomized controlled trials showed that devil's claw as a powder (containing 60mg of the active constituent harpagoside) was moderately effective in relieving osteoarthritis of the spine, hip and knee.[37]

Both varieties of devil's claw are also often recommended for natural pain relief of gout.

Suggested daily dosage: 750mg with at least 3 per cent harpagoside three times a day (or the equivalent of 9g of crude plant material) over at least two to three months

WARNING: Devil's claw can, apparently, interfere with diabetes medications, blood thinners and other prescription drugs.

Guggul

Although Ayurveda, the traditional system of healthcare in India, offers many remedies for osteoarthritis, one of the key ingredients found in Ayurvedic arthritis medicine is guggul, a resin of the herb *Commiphora mukul*. According to one study, patients taking guggul significantly improved in pain and mobility after one month.[38]

Suggested daily dosage: 500mg taken with food

Traditional Chinese herbs

Traditional Chinese Medicine has specific herbs for arthritis too, and claims startling success with them. In a randomized clinical study, two formulas called Shu Guan Wen Jing and Shu Guan Qing Luo were recently reported to actually 'cure' over 50 per cent of rheumatoid arthritis patients – with no side effects.[39]

Another Chinese herbal medicine, Lei gong teng (thunder god vine or 'three-wing nut'; *Tripterygium wilfordii Hook F*), works against rheumatoid arthritis by inhibiting pro-inflammatory agents in the body, such as tumour necrosis factor (TNF)-alpha and cyclooxygenase (COX)-2.[40]

Suggested daily dosage for Chinese herbs: 180–360mg, as directed by an experienced practitioner

Yucca

A herbal remedy made from the yucca plant, which is native to Mexico, has also been shown to be helpful in easing the symptoms of RA.[41] *Yucca schidigera* is a medicinal plant native to Mexico. According to folk medicine, yucca extracts have anti-arthritic and anti-inflammatory effects, largely because it is a potent source of steroidal saponins, which have powerful anti-parasitical activity. Some researchers believe that the herb works by suppressing intestinal bugs that play a role in inflammation of joints, as with RA. Yucca also contains polyphenols, including resveratrol, which themselves have anti-inflammatory effects.[42]

Cayenne cream

Also called capsaicin cream, this is an extract of cayenne pepper that can ease many types of chronic pain when regularly applied to the skin. The spice comes from dried hot peppers and alleviates pain by depleting the body's supply of substance P, a chemical component of nerve cells that transmit pain signals to the brain.

In one study, a capsaicin plaster was significantly better than a placebo in patients with chronic back pain.[43] Research has shown this approach to reduce pain and tenderness by up to 40 per cent in people with osteoarthritis of the hands.[44]

Willow bark

Willow bark, or *Salix alba* as it is known scientifically, is chemically related to aspirin, and appears to provide short-term relief for patients with lower back pain.[45]

||||||||||||||||||||||||||||||||||||||||||||

Chapter 10

SUPER SUPPLEMENTS FOR ARTHRITIS

While alternative therapies offer much to a sufferer of arthritis in any of its forms, there's a great deal that you can also do for yourself. Besides a radical change of diet, a low-impact exercise programme and the introduction of vitamin and mineral supplements into your daily regime can result in enormous benefits, just as they have for many thousands of others before you. That said, it's advisable to work with a qualified, experienced nutritional therapist on any major changes to your diet or before beginning supplementation.

Below you'll find guidance on the best-researched supplements shown to have good effects in terms of lowering inflammation and improving joint function. But do bear in mind that these are not magic bullets. They mainly work as part of a holistic treatment that includes discovering the causes of your inflammation and incorporating the right diet, exercise and mind–body medicine.

The following list of bio-compounds, herbs, enzymes, minerals, vitamins and plant extracts comes from a wide variety of sources and geographic locations, including Indian Ayruvedic medicine, Traditional Chinese Medicine, and traditional folk medicine from a wide variety of countries. The first section in this chapter is dedicated to supplements that directly treat arthritis and its symptoms. The second section offers a list of natural painkillers. However, a number of these supplements do both.

They work best in combination with all the lifestyle and mind–body suggestions put forward in this book.

Glucosamine and chondroitin

These two unusual, naturally occurring compounds, sold as nutritional supplements, have been revolutionizing alternative treatments for arthritis. Both substances are of major importance in assisting the growth of cartilage, the spongy material that covers the ends of bones in the joints and protects them from wear.

Glucosamine is the major building block of proteoglycans, the large molecules in cartilage that give it its elastic and protective properties, maintaining joint lubrication and flexibility by trapping water in the cartilage matrix. Chondroitin, an even larger cartilage molecule, helps to maintain joint fluidity, while slowing cartilage destruction and helping with its repair.[1] Glucosamine works by stopping the breakdown of proteoglycans and by rebuilding damaged cartilage. Clinical trials show that it appears to be a natural anti-inflammatory as well.

Chondroitin helps reduce cartilage loss in as little as six months after starting supplements.[2] A recent review of the evidence concluded that oral chondroitin sulphate 'is a valuable and safe symptomatic treatment for OA [osteoarthritis] disease.' Interestingly, 800mg/day had nearly the same effects as 1200mg/day in one study.[3] It's often recommended that chondroitin be taken in combination with glucosamine. One theory is that both these agents work by improving the quality of the synovial fluid between the joints.[4]

Overall evidence for their healing effect is impressive. One of the most comprehensive trials was an international study on more than 200 patients with osteoarthritis of the knee. They were given either 1500mg of glucosamine or a placebo daily over the course of three years. Double-blind assessment showed that, while there was the predictable deterioration of the joints in the placebo group, the glucosamine group's joints remained intact. There was a corresponding improvement in pain and joint mobility, with no significant side effects. The researchers were impressed by glucosamine's 'long-term combined structure-modifying and symptom-modifying effects'. This therefore appears to be one of the first natural substances to have a genuine effect on the disease itself.[5]

This study proved to be a breakthrough for supporters of nutritional supplements, since medical commentary accompanying publication of the study included the admission that doctors must begin to 'accommodate the possibility that many nutritional products may have valuable therapeutic effects'.[6]

In another study 80 patients with osteoarthritis were given either 500mg of glucosamine sulphate or a placebo three times a day. While symptoms decreased in both groups, those receiving glucosamine had a significantly greater reduction in symptoms compared with placebo – 73 versus 41 per cent. Furthermore, a sample of cartilage from the placebo group, looked at under electron microscopy, showed evidence of osteoarthritis, whereas samples from the treated patients looked more like healthy cartilage.[7]

The medical community has generally disparaged these supplements, pointing to studies showing glucosamine to have no effects – trials that have since been criticized as having serious flaws and poor study design – while failing to take seriously an ever-rising tide of studies that have been conducted properly and that clearly demonstrate glucosamine's effectiveness.

More recently, glucosamine has been compared with conventional NSAIDs. In a recent trial of 600 osteoarthritis patients conducted all over Europe, a chondroitin and glucosamine combination was pitted against celecoxib, one of the major COX-2 inhibitor drugs. The supplements worked as well as the COX-2 drug: both groups saw a more than 50 per cent reduction in joint swelling, with similar improvements in joint pain, stiffness and function after six months.[8]

Moreover, when 54 trials involving more than 16,000 patients were pooled together, glucosamine and chondroitin, either alone or together, were shown to be just as effective as celecoxib for relieving painful knee osteoarthritis, although only the supplement combination significantly improved joint function and led to a marked improvement in the knee-joint space narrowing commonly seen in the condition.[9]

Chondroitin alone also beat celecoxib at reducing cartilage loss in knee osteoarthritis, although both pills were equally good at easing pain and improving function.[10]

Supplements vs ibuprofen

Glucosamine also wins out against ibuprofen as a painkiller for treating osteoarthritis. In one study, patients with temporomandibular joint (TMJ) disorders treated with glucosamine had less pain and less difficulty opening their mouths than those treated with the common painkiller.[11]

Although they take a little longer to work, glucosamine and chondroitin deliver as much painkilling and anti-inflammatory action as the standard NSAIDs, and even actually improve joint function and reduce cartilage loss – all without serious side effects.

The effects of glucosamine sulphate are known to improve over time. So, if you wish to try it, give it at least three months.

Suggested daily dosages:

Glucosamine sulphate: up to 3,200mg

Chondroitin: up to 3,600mg

Collagen hydrolysate

Collagen hydrolysate, a gelatin, has been shown to be successful in the treatment of osteoarthritis and other joint disorders in arthritis patients12 and to halt its progression in mice. [13]

Suggested daily dosage: up to 1,200mg

CH-Alpha

CH-Alpha is a registered product whose main active ingredients are hydrolyzed collagen, extracts of *Zingiber officinale* (ginger) root,

Boswellia serrata, *Rosa canina* fruit (rosehip), and vitamin C. It comes in oral and gel applications. The gel contains *Arnica montana* and sunflower seed oil as well.

Several studies have been done on CH-Alpha.[14] In one of them, 100 athletes at the Rhein-Ruhr Olympic Training Facilities in Essen, Germany, were each given 10g of CH-Alpha daily for 12 weeks after having their movement and pain levels initially assessed. The patients taking the supplement showed significant improvements in all areas of pain and mobility, compared to initial assessments.[15]

Hyaluronic acid

Hyaluronic acid is a fluid carbohydrate and another of the building blocks of cartilage, and taken as a supplement it appears to decrease the production of enzymes that damage healthy cartilage tissue and also interfere with pain signals. When injected directly into the knee joint, it can help improve function.[16] It can also be taken orally. Based on animal studies (which, of course, may not apply to humans), this appears to work best when taken in a preparation that includes phospholipids.[17] And in a study of people, those with osteoarthritis of the knee had less pain and overall improvement in function with oral daily supplements taken for eight weeks.[18]

Hyaluronic acid is sometimes injected directly into the joint to act as a lubricant – a process referred to as 'viscosupplementation'. Recent studies have shown that this is effective for osteoarthritis of the knee and ankle, with patients reporting significant improvements in pain and function.[19]

Suggested daily dosage: 40mg

MSM (methylsulphonylmethane)

A source of bioavailable sulphur found in the tissues and fluids of all plants, animals and humans, MSM can reduce pain and swelling, and stop the destruction of joints by scavenging the free radicals that cause inflammation. It's been shown to reduce pain and improve function when taken orally for at least 12 weeks.[20]

Suggested daily dosage: up to 1,200mg in divided dosages

SAM-e (S-adenosylmethionine)

This naturally occurring compound, present in virtually every tissue and fluid in the body, is known to be a powerful anti-inflammatory. Besides reducing pain, it can improve joint function and ease stiffness.[21] Double-blind trials show that SAMe (1,200mg/day) reduces pain, stiffness and swelling in osteoarthritis sufferers better than a placebo, and with the same effectiveness as painkilling drugs such as ibuprofen and naproxen.[22]

SAMe appears to stimulate the production of cartilage and, although researchers don't know exactly why, it may even reduce inflammation, influence cartilage synthesis and survival, and boost the production of antioxidants.[23]

Suggested daily dosage: Up to 1,200mg in divided dosages

Avocado/soya bean unsaponifiable (ASU) oils

These special oil mixtures can promote cartilage repair and reduce circulating levels of pro-inflammatory cytokines, so improving function and reducing pain as well as the need to take NSAIDs.[24]

Vitamins and minerals

If arthritis is already present, the antioxidants vitamins C and E and the mineral selenium have been shown to reduce the pain of rheumatoid arthritis.[25] Rheumatoid arthritis sufferers have been found to benefit from supplements of vitamin E, beta-carotene and selenium[26] and to be deficient in zinc.[27]

Suggested daily dosage: Doctors such as Dr John Mansfield recommend that patients supplement with a good multivitamin/mineral, a B complex vitamin formula with at least 25mg of B5 (pantothenic acid) and B3 (niacinamide), plus zinc (50mg), selenium (200mcg), and vitamin D (2,000–3,000IU) if you're deficient in it.

Vitamin C is essential for collagen synthesis; taking megadoses of 1g or more can reduce the risk of cartilage loss by 70 per cent.[28] Vitamin E can also help to reduce pain – and may even have an anti-inflammatory effect.[29] So take both vitamins together. Dosages of 1,200 to 1,800IU per day of vitamin E can significantly decrease joint pain.[30]

Suggested daily dosages:

Vitamin C: 1–3g

Vitamin E: 1,200–1,800IU

B vitamins

Individual B vitamins have been shown to help increase movement and reduce pain in arthritis sufferers. Niacinamide, a form of vitamin B3, reduces inflammation, increases joint mobility and reduces the need for painkilling first-line anti-inflammatories that osteoarthritis sufferers need to take.[31]

B5 (pantothenic acid) and B3 (niacinamide) have been shown to be beneficial at doses of 25mg. Vitamin B12 and folic acid have been shown to help improve grip strength in patients with arthritis of the hands and fingers.[32] For rheumatoid arthritis sufferers taking methotrexate, folic acid supplements can reduce the toxicity of this powerful immunosuppressant drug.[33]

Suggested daily dosages: The B vitamins should be taken within a balanced B-complex supplement and should not be taken at night.

B5: 25mg

Niacinamide: from 900mg to 4g a day in divided doses – but only under medical supervision as high levels can cause glucose intolerance and liver damage

B12 and folic acid: 800mcg each

Boron

Boron, a natural mineral, has been used for years as a supplement for arthritis – without side effects.[34] It's also given for osteoporosis. Boron given to rats and chicks has increased bone strength. However, clinical studies are needed to clarify boron's effects in humans.[35]

What Doctors Don't Tell You panel member Dr Melvyn Werbach suggests that, as the minimum daily allowance for boron still isn't established, patients should increase their consumption of boron-rich foods (vegetables such as soybeans, cabbage, lettuce and peas;

fruits such as apples, dates, raisins and prunes; and nuts, especially almonds, hazelnuts and peanuts).

Magnesium oil

When magnesium levels fall, there's a marked increase in inflammatory cytokines, along with increased levels of histamine – at least in rodents.[36] Many people claim that spraying magnesium oil regularly onto the skin and rubbing it into painful areas has brought relief for the joint pain associated with arthritic conditions.

Copper

If you have RA, consider getting your copper levels tested, as sufferers are often deficient in this mineral. Supplement only under the guidance of a qualified, experienced professional.

Supplements for gout

Supplements that may help with gout include fish oils, the B vitamins (particularly folic acid), vitamin E and vitamin C.

The vitamin D connection

As we've seen, many of the above supplements that serve as remedies for arthritis also work as effective pain relievers, and one of the most interesting natural supplements to consider for pain relief of arthritis is vitamin D.

In a nationwide study of nearly 7,000 adults from across Britain, scientists at the Institute of Child Health in London discovered a link between low levels of vitamin D and chronic widespread pain. Although the findings weren't significant for men, in women the prevalence of this chronic pain varied according to vitamin D concentrations. Women with vitamin D levels between 75 and 99nmol/l – the range deemed necessary for bone health – had the lowest rates of pain: just over 8 per cent. In contrast, in women who had levels less than 25nmol/l, pain rates were nearly doubled at 14.4 per cent.[37]

Similar results were reported in an American study. Mayo Clinic researchers in Rochester, Minnesota, found a connection between inadequate vitamin D levels and the amount of opiate-containing medication taken by patients suffering from chronic pain. Those who had low vitamin D levels were taking much higher doses of pain medication – nearly twice as much – as those whose levels were adequate. Moreover, they reported poorer physical functioning and poorer overall perception of health.[38]

Although these two studies aren't proof that a lack of vitamin D causes chronic pain, they do contribute to a mounting body of evidence suggesting an important role for this vitamin in pain control. Indeed, according to an extensive review of the research so far, inadequate vitamin D has been linked to a long list of painful maladies, including bone and joint pain, muscle aches, fibromyalgia, rheumatic disorders, osteoarthritis and other complaints.[39]

Much of the research has focused on chronic musculoskeletal-related pain. Indeed, the review's author, Dr Stewart Leavitt, identified 22 clinical studies investigating vitamin D status in patients with this sort of pain. Across these studies overall, an average of around 70 per cent of patients with chronic musculoskeletal pain were found to be deficient in the vitamin.

The evidence also shows that supplementing with vitamin D can lead to a dramatic reduction in pain. In more than 350 people with chronic back pain, vitamin D therapy led to symptomatic improvement in 95 per cent – and in 100 per cent of those with the most severe vitamin D deficiencies.[40]

According to Leavitt, vitamin D deficiency can contribute to musculoskeletal pain by causing hypocalcaemia – low levels of circulating calcium – which 'sets in motion a cascade of biochemical reactions negatively affecting bone metabolism and health'. One of these reactions is an increase in parathyroid hormone (PTH), which can impair proper bone mineralization, causing a spongy bone matrix to form in the skeleton. This matrix absorbs fluid and expands, causing the resultant ballooning pressure to trigger pain in the tissues overlying the bones, since sensory pain fibres are abundant in these tissues.

In addition, vitamin D deficiency can contribute to pain in other ways. Several studies cited by Leavitt in his report found that vitamin D may play a role in non-musculoskeletal pain syndromes, including neuropathy, migraine headaches and inflammatory autoimmune conditions such as inflammatory bowel disease.

Whatever the mechanism involved, the data suggest that checking for vitamin D deficiency – and correcting it – should be an important part of chronic pain management.

Sunlight is the best source of this vitamin but, as most of us don't get enough of it this way, Leavitt recommends taking – with the supervision of a qualified practitioner – a daily supplement of 2,000IU of vitamin D3 (cholecalciferol), along with a daily multivitamin that includes calcium and 400–800IU of vitamin D. He notes that it may take up to nine months to experience the maximum effect of such a regimen.

Other nutrients for chronic pain

Besides vitamin D, other nutrients may be beneficial for people with chronic pain. These include proteolytic (digestive) enzymes such as bromelain, as suggested in the chapter on gut problems (*see page 83*), and amino acids such as d-phenylalanine and l-tryptophan. Taken with a glucosamine/chrondroitin sulphate combination, proteolytic enzymes are known to be as effective as NSAIDs for inflammatory conditions such as arthritis of the shoulder or knee,[41] while amino acids appear to increase pain tolerance.[42]

For natural pain relief of gout, varieties of the herb devil's claw (*Harpagophytum procumbens* or *H. radix*) have often been recommended, based on evidence for its effectiveness in various forms of arthritis.[43]

Alternatively, try homeopathic remedies (*see page 129*.)

Chapter 11

NON-SURGICAL SURGERY

Joe Maroon's knee was giving way to osteoarthritis. After years of running, biking and swimming, Maroon's cartilage had significantly deteriorated, causing constant pain. Doctors told the 63-year-old triathlete that he needed knee replacement surgery, but as a doctor himself, a neurosurgeon at the University of Pittsburgh, he was well aware of what that might entail. Had he been just a few years younger, his doctor might not have even presented that option, since artificial hips or knees wear out after about a decade and then need to be replaced again: hence, doctors like their patients to defer that first operation for as long as possible.

The only alternative seemed to be a lifetime of steroid injections and the overwhelming likelihood of having to end his competitive sporting activities.

During his years of trying to figure out how to deal with this worsening condition, Maroon chanced upon the Centeno-Schultz Clinic's orthopaedic alternative, Regenexx™, to heal damaged joints. Maroon was impressed enough to investigate.

Owner and medical director of the Centeno-Schultz Clinic, in Broomfield, a suburb of Denver, Colorado, Dr Chris Centeno, a 51-year-old pain-management specialist, has pioneered a technique that uses the patient's own stem cells to restore damaged tissue – cartilage, bone, ligaments and tendons – largely ending the need for surgery.

After some of Joe's stem cells were extracted from his bone marrow, they were cultured and so multiplied in the lab over several weeks before being re-injected into his damaged knee. The result was such a reduction of pain that Maroon, by that time aged 68, was able to compete in the Ironman Hawai'i triathlon six months later.

Most joint issues are caused by deterioration of cartilage (which cushions the movement of bones, especially in the hips and knees), usually owing to inflammation; and as cartilage is poorly supplied with blood, it ordinarily doesn't regenerate.

Medicine makes tacit recognition of this fact with the few alternatives to joint replacement it offers. Surgery to repair cartilage either attempts to 'injure' it to prompt the bone beneath it to initiate a repair response, or else chunks of healthy cartilage are implanted into areas of damage as a form of tissue engineering.[1]

Cartilage repair has a spotty record of success,[2] since transplants are often destroyed by the body's own natural inflammatory response.

After the turn of the millennium, Centeno, profoundly dissatisfied with the state of orthopaedic medicine and its reliance on steroids and surgery, became interested in animal research on stem cells,[3] and wondered whether it might apply to people too. The research was showing that when damaged joints were injected with the animal's own stem cells, the cells, as if responding to some hidden blueprint, would differentiate into the appropriate tissues required to heal the damage. Even more encouraging, the tissue continued to do its repair job over time.

Centeno wanted to test whether the ready supply of malleable mesenchymal stem cells (MSCs), which are already likely to turn into bone, cartilage and connective tissue cells, present in the bone marrow of most patients, could be used to rebuild damaged joints. His revelation came when he realized that adding a solution of the patient's own blood platelets to the brew would 'supercharge' the MSCs to replicate and also to differentiate into more cartilage and bone to repair the joint. Centeno partnered with Dr John Schultz, an orthopaedic specialist and anesthesiologist, and the Centeno-Schultz Clinic opened its doors in Broomfield.

Early on, Centeno had also decided to substantiate the clinic's work by carrying out painstaking research and follow-up on all their patients and publishing the findings, ultimately spending $500,000 of his own funds on mainly research programmes. So far, Centeno has carried out more research on stem-cell orthopaedic repair than any other research centre.

M is for mesenchymal

Stem cells are nothing less than shape-shifters – precursor cells that go on to differentiate into whatever kind of cell tissue is required. They have most controversially been harvested from human embryos and adipose (fat) tissue, but those with the best record of success and safety for treating joint problems are the so-called mesenchymal stem cells (MSCs), found in large numbers in bone marrow tissue. Although other clinics use stem cells from adipose tissue in joints, Centeno believes that MSCs are considered superior because these cells are already partially committed to becoming bone, muscle, ligament or tendon, are easily harvested from bone marrow and reproduce rapidly, making them ideal candidates for repairing those very structures. According to Centeno, under certain conditions MSCs can be prompted to differentiate into the specific sort of tissue needed; when implanted into affected joints, these cells work to repair cartilage and bone, and the connective tissues in between. Indeed, there's even evidence they can protect against inflammation-related tissue damage and have the ability to modulate autoimmune responses too.[4]

In 2008, he published the results of an early trial for his procedure. His guinea pig was a man who'd suffered for years from knee pain that hadn't improved with surgery. Centeno harvested MSCs from the patient's hip bone, then multiplied and 'boosted' them by culturing the cells with factors from the patient's blood platelets. After a few days, he injected this brew into the patient's knee.

The results were unequivocal. Just a month after the procedure, the patient's knee cartilage surface area had expanded by more than 20 per cent, and the joint meniscus – the cushiony cartilaginous pad that bears the brunt of the thighbone's weight – was also 29 per cent larger after six months.[5] The patient's previously limited range of motion was now nearly normal and his pain level, formerly assessed as 4 out of a possible 10, had plummeted to 0.4.

The clinic's database

In the intervening six years, Centeno and his colleagues (including doctors he has trained around the world) have performed some 10,000 procedures on all manner of orthopaedic and soft-tissue injuries, hundreds of them involving patients with diseased knee and hip joints. The results are impressive – even more so because his patients continue to improve over months, even years.

Recently, Centeno's own registry data showed that, of 221 overweight and older patients with knee arthritis, 80 per cent recorded more than a 25 per cent improvement after the operation, with an average of nearly 60 per cent improvement after two years. And of 999 middle-aged people who were only slightly overweight, the figures showed that 90 per cent reported a more than 50 per cent improvement, with more than 70 per cent average improvement after four years.

Although the results for hip pain are not as spectacular, more than 60 per cent of such patients still reported more than 25 per cent pain relief, with an average improvement of 42 per cent in patients under 55 (22 per cent in those older than 55).

Puzzling over why hip patients don't do as well as knee patients, the Regenexx team studied their post-treatment registry and discovered that a patient's total range of hip motion was connected to outcome success: the poorer the range of motion, the poorer the outcome of the standard treatment (whereby the patient's own stem cells are not cultured, but just injected back in).

Nevertheless, both hip and knee stem-cell patients fare well when compared with joint replacement patients. According to an independent comparison made by American orthopaedic surgeon Dr Mitch Sheinkof, patients getting hip replacements showed a greater improvement in the Harris hip test (which measures pain and movement ability), but Regenexx patients enjoyed a better range of motion and a better overall risk/benefit ratio, as the stem-cell procedure is far less invasive and carries far less risk. Some 73 per cent of the hip Regenexx patients were able to return to sporting activities. Knee patients in particular show greater overall functional improvement.

In 2011, Centeno and his team published a safety and complications report on 339 patients, most of whom had arthritis of the knee and all of whom had been told they needed knee replacements. After receiving the stem-cell Regenexx treatment, only 4.1 per cent of these patients went on to get an artificial knee, while the rest did well enough with the Regenexx treatment to avoid surgery.

Not surprisingly, Centeno has been singled out by the US Food and Drug Administration (FDA), largely because his work appears to fall outside the agency's jurisdiction. Stem-cell therapy not only threatens to revolutionize orthopaedic medicine as we know it, but also threatens to wipe away some of the £30 billion pain-management drug business and ultimately to rock the foundations of FDA control of the entire drugs marketplace.

The FDA has visited the Colorado clinic many times – sifting through Centeno's laboratory 'as if it were a mass drug manufacturing factory', as he puts it. In August 2010, the Center for Biologics Evaluation and Research, a division of the FDA, filed an injunction, ordering his clinic to stop culturing patients' stem cells. In response, he filed for multiple temporary restraining orders simultaneously in Denver and in Washington, DC. The FDA then issued another injunction against the clinic, whereupon Centeno abandoned the restraining orders and promptly countersued the FDA for interfering with his trade.

The FDA maintains that extracting, manipulating and culturing a person's stem cells constitutes a 'cultured drug product' not unlike culturing an antibiotic. In 2012, in an attempt to control this new medical technique, the FDA ruled that your own stem cells should now be considered a 'drug' subject to the agency's control.

The FDA's ruling was upheld in a court case, even though Centeno argued that 'stem cells are body parts and not the property of the government or Big Pharma'. 'What we're doing in our medical practice,' claims his partner Schultz, 'is no different, in principle, than a fertility clinic that uses *in vitro* fertilization'. At the time, the ruling meant that the clinic could only treat those parts of the body that receive enough blood flow to benefit from an ordinary stem cell injection – harvested from the hip and immediately injected into the damaged joint.

As Centeno and Schultz are no longer able to culture stem cells within the USA, they were forced to move that part of their practice to the Cayman Islands, which is outside FDA jurisdiction. In most cases this isn't an impediment to the work in the Colorado clinic, as 90 per cent of their practice concerns situations where patients can benefit from having their existing MSCs harvested and injected back in. Any patients with problems requiring a larger batch of stem cells will now travel to the clinic in the Caymans, funds permitting.

Possibly because research has shown that the native stem cells in the hips aren't as robust as those in knees and have less of an inbuilt repair mechanism, older hip patients tend to do far better with cultured stem cells than ones just taken out of the patient's bone marrow and re-injected back in.

In October 2013, the FDA published a rider to clarify its initial ruling, allowing work like Centeno's to carry on so long as the harvested stem cells are returned to the patient without too much manipulation and as part of the 'same' procedure. This amounted to a cautious stamp of approval for the clinic to carry on its work with damaged joints, using a procedure that simply harvests MSCs from the hipbone, then purifies them and injects them directly into the damaged joint.

A number of other orthopaedic specialists are also using stem-cell technology, albeit without the scientific monitoring or published data that Centeno brings to his work.

Despite the FDA's challenges, Centeno remains confident that the sheer weight of evidence of the safety and success of his procedure will speak for itself – and prevail.

Can stem cells cause cancer?

It's well known that injecting embryo-derived stem cells into a patient can cause tumours to develop. For this reason, Centeno and his team as well as others have kept careful follow-up data on patients receiving MSCs for orthopaedic purposes. Several years ago, Centeno published follow-up data on more than 300 patients who'd been tracked for up to four years, many of whom were later scanned for procedure-related problems, including tumours.[6] This is the largest study of its kind and the first of a set of similar studies. No cancerous growths or formations were found.

In a separate study, Japanese researchers went even further, following 45 patients who'd received MSC transplants to repair cartilage, for more than 11 years. They could find no evidence of either tumours or infections.

Chapter 12

LIFESTYLE FOR HEALTHY JOINTS

Doctors treating soldiers during World War Two began to notice that their patients had different reactions to the same kinds of wounds: some asked for more pain medication than others. For some their injuries translated into an attitude of 'Hooray! I survived and I'm going home!' For others it was: 'Now I'm a cripple and will never amount to anything.' Unsurprisingly, it was usually the latter, more depressed, group that needed more pain medication. From these experiences, the doctors began to appreciate that a person's general mind-set about injury or illness played a crucial role in the amount of pain he or she experienced.[1]

Since those days, scientists now reckon that a positive mental attitude could be one of the key elements to curbing – even possibly reversing – the pain of arthritis, which is why taking a more holistic, mind–body approach to treatment and healing for all diseases, including arthritis, is so effective.

Many alternative 'body therapies' also involve some element of the mind or harnessing the healing powers of the 'life force' or *chi*. Others, such as chiropractic and the Alexander Technique, can improve posture. Some of the major body/mind therapies are reviewed here, as well as some simple 'self-help' things you can do, such as low-impact exercise and meditation.

Hypnotherapy

Hypnosis is a well-known and accepted psychological technique that slows down the brain's cycles, inducing more theta or alpha brain waves in the patient, both of which indicate highly suggestible states of consciousness. While the subject is in this comfortable receptive state, the therapist introduces suggestions to bring about changes in physical, mental and emotional behaviour, as well as subjective experiences of perception and sensation.

Hypnosis appears to help people with chronic pain manage both the intensity of the pain they feel and their emotional response to that pain, and to provide them with a sense of involvement in their own treatment.[2]

One scientific review of good studies on hypnosis found it to be effective for chronic pain. The combined results of 18 studies indicated that the average person treated with hypnosis obtained greater pain relief than 75 per cent of those given conventional care or no treatment at all.[3]

In another review, researchers examined the use of hypnosis for chronic headache, lower back pain, temporomandibular joint (TMJ) pain and pain resulting from cancer, as well as acute pain related to fibromyalgia, osteoarthritis and disability. Hypnotherapy consistently provided greater relief than conventional or no treatment, leading them to the conclusion that 'hypnotic treatment for chronic pain results in significant reductions in perceived pain that maintain for at least several months, and possibly longer'.[4]

Doctors also report their own experience that hypnosis is highly useful for pain management in both acute and chronic situations because it enables patients to control the intensity of their pain as well as the emotional intensity accompanying symptoms.[5]

A further bonus of hypnosis is that it's almost always a benign treatment, with little risk of negative side effects. What 'side effects' do occur are overwhelmingly positive, including a greater sense of control over pain, greater overall feelings of well-being, and less tension, stress and anxiety.[6]

Biofeedback

With biofeedback, electrical sensors are attached to the body that measure such things as heart rate, muscle tension, body temperature and brainwave activity. The patterns are displayed on a video monitor to help you receive information (feedback) about your body (bio). Following the visual feedback from the sensors, a patient can quickly learn how to create subtle changes in their body – such as relaxing specific muscles – in order to achieve specific results, such as lowering blood pressure or reducing muscle tension or pain.

A non-invasive technique with no side effects, biofeedback has been successfully used to treat a range of problems, including chronic pain, eating disorders, PTSD (post-traumatic stress disorder), migraines, phobias, sexual disorders, urinary incontinence, addictions and numerous other conditions.

A number of studies have found biofeedback to be more effective than conventional treatments for chronic pain.[7]

Emotional Freedom Technique (EFT)

This simple process, which entails gently tapping on particular acupuncture points while repeating certain relevant phrases aloud, addresses underlying emotional issues and unresolved subconscious traumas that can trigger any number of health issues – including arthritis. Favoured by some alternative health practitioners and psychologists, EFT has been used with excellent success to treat patients with severe low back pain and other health and pain-related issues.

Manipulation-based techniques

A number of primary hands-on manipulation techniques, which focus primarily on physiological structure – adjusting the position and alignment of bones and joints, and manipulating soft tissues, thus aiding the circulatory and lymphatic systems – are used to address arthritis pain. All these methods employ highly individualized approaches that address the unique needs of each patient.

Chiropractic

Chiropractic manipulation – specifically, spinal manipulation therapy (SMT) – is highly effective for chronic back-pain patients. Studies show that it has significant benefits compared with sham manipulations and other more conventional treatments that can be ineffective or even harmful, such as bed rest and traction.[8] SMT is also used to treat a wide variety of other painful conditions, including fibromyalgia, carpal tunnel syndrome and migraine and in general is found to be more effective than conventional treatments in relieving pain and disability generally.[9]

However, chiropractic involves more than adjusting the spine, neck and other joints. For people suffering from rheumatoid arthritis there are a number of ways it can minimize damage, slow the pace of the condition and ease pain. Among other techniques in the chiropractic arsenal for arthritis are:

Ultrasound therapy using sound waves to help reduce swelling and decrease pain and stiffness

Trigger-point therapy, which is the application of gentle pressure to a specific muscles where a patient experiences pain (similar to acupressure)

Low-level or 'cold laser' therapy, which uses a non-heat-producing laser to reduce inflammation

Therapeutic exercises and stretches – physical activities designed specifically for people with RA to promote strength and endurance; they can be done in the office or at home

Massage

Massage therapy, which usually focuses on soft tissues, including muscles, tendons and ligaments, also helps alleviate chronic pain. Although there are dozens of different massage techniques, the most well studied include Swedish massage and deep-tissue massage point therapy. In a comprehensive review by the Cochrane Collaboration, massage was shown to be more effective than numerous other treatment methods, including joint mobilization, physical therapy, acupuncture and relaxation therapy for the treatment of lower back pain. Even better was the longevity of its beneficial effects, which were shown to last at least a year beyond the end of the treatment.[10]

In another study of patients suffering from chronic pain, massage therapy was at least as effective as standard medical care in the short term. Even more importantly, after three months comparing traditional treatment with massage, only those in the massage group still showed significant improvement.[11]

Massage is thought to work because it promotes better circulation of blood and lymph flow to affected areas, but it's also been discovered that massage may raise serotonin levels produced by the brain, thus modulating the body's pain-control system. Another possibility is that the deep relaxation massage acts to aid restorative sleep, which reduces levels of substance P, a brain chemical associated with pain.[12]

Copper

Wearing copper bracelets for arthritis sounds like ancient folklore, but it appears to have begun only in the 1970s. At the time, doctors tended to dismiss it out of hand, claiming that the benefits were imagined and that any pain relief was due to the natural ebb and flow of the disease.

Then, according to one controlled study whereby 300 people with arthritis were given real copper bracelets, look-alike fake ones or none at all, the idea 'appeared to have some therapeutic value'.[13] The results seemed to fit with an earlier finding, that arthritis patients excrete abnormally high amounts of copper in their urine and may have altered copper metabolism,[14] as well as more recent evidence.[15]

So, does the bracelet work because it's acting as a source of copper? According to Australian rheumatologist, Dr Ray Walker, author of the 1976 study, the answer is a categorical 'yes. Copper,' he claims, 'when in contact with the skin, interacts with human sweat (sometimes seen as a green deposit under the bracelet) and is thus absorbed through the skin. Think of a bracelet as a "time-release" source of copper.'

The reason the bracelets work is less mysterious than it seems. We know that the worse the RA, the more elevated the blood levels of copper. Copper concentrations in the synovial fluid (found in the joints) in RA sufferers are also three times those of non-sufferers. But the rise in these copper concentrations leads to a drop in levels of copper in the liver and other copper-storing tissues. These localized copper deficiencies lead to an increase of iron in these tissues, which may help to cause RA.

Using copper bracelets restores some of this lost copper. In the study of 300 patients, each bracelet lost copper while being worn. Interestingly, the very low incidence of RA in pre-industrial Europe has been put down to the use of copper cooking utensils and plates.[16]

Copper is also effective for pain relief. Anthroposophical medicine – a holistic system of medicine developed by 19th-century educator, philosopher and social reformer Rudolf Steiner – had many years of success with a copper ointment used for pain in RA.[17] Copper may also have an anti-inflammatory effect related to its ability to form selective antioxidants.[18]

It also may work through the action of superoxide dismutase, an enzyme that breaks down superoxide radicals through a reaction catalysed in the enzyme by copper and zinc.[19]

Spa therapy

Also known as balneotherapy, spa therapy is another approach with ancient roots. Bathing in mineral waters such as the Dead Sea or in thermal waters in hot springs at temperatures of around 34ºC (93ºF) can significantly relieve arthritis pain from a variety of arthritic conditions.[20] Balneotherapy may involve either hot or cold water and water massage from jets and moving water. Medicinal clays applied to the body as a mud bath are also frequently used.

Exercise for arthritis prevention

Regular moderate exercise is essential for retarding joint deterioration. Activities that don't put stress on joints but strengthen surrounding bones, muscles and ligaments are effective for dealing with many types of arthritis and may also be preventative. If you know your ligaments are looser than normal, good choices include cycling, walking and swimming. Just avoid weight-bearing or high-impact exercises.

Moderate exercise can help keep your body healthy into older age. Even elderly patients with existing problems such as heart disease and arthritis see improvements in their condition once they've started a healthy exercise regime. In one study, patients over 60 with osteoarthritis of the knee noticed improvements in their condition and mobility after 18 months of aerobic exercise. Overall, older people who regularly exercise have stronger hearts, better circulation, stronger bones, better balance, less pain, better sleep quality, sharper minds and a reduced risk of many cancers.[21]

Aerobic exercise

Aerobic exercise of all kinds – dance, biking, swimming – is excellent for stress management and, done properly, helps mitigate the effects of all forms of arthritis, including fibromyalgia. Aerobic exercise has been shown to decrease pain levels, lift depression, aid sleep and increase overall energy.

While there seems to be little evidence of a risk of arthritis in male runners, the same doesn't hold true for women. A study of some 80 former élite British female athletes – mostly runners – found they had a greater risk of osteoarthritis in the hips and knees than did non-athletes, particularly where the knee joins the upper leg bone, or femur.[22]

The researchers concluded that weight-bearing sports activity in women is associated with a two-to-threefold increased risk of osteoarthritis (especially the presence of osteophytes) in the knees and hips.

Whether or not you'll suffer permanent knee injury has to do with another important consideration: joint alignment. One of the greatest health risks from sports, which affects both genders and can lead to osteoarthritis, is injury to the ligaments that attach to the knee. Evidence shows that distance runners may risk developing lax knee joints due to loosening of the ligaments that attach to and support the knee. A loose knee is, in essence, a wobbly one that's more prone to joint displacement.[23] The main ligaments involved are the anterior and posterior cruciate ligaments, two finger-sized pieces of tissue that crisscross within the knee joint and support the joint as well as allow it to rotate comfortably.

At present the statistics for female athletes are sobering. Women involved in running and jumping sports are four to eight times more likely to do their knees in than men are. In the USA, women collegiate athletes suffer some 10,000 knee injuries a year. Several theories suggest that anatomy predisposes women to running injuries: the wider pelvis exaggerates the angle of the knee when running and moving, and female hormones – present in knee ligaments – cause them to be naturally more stretchy than those in men. The lesser leg strength of women and slower reaction times can also increase the risk of injury.

With three times the hamstring strength of women, men are built to stride faster. The bony space in the femur through which the anterior cruciate ligament passes is also smaller in women than in men, leading to a smaller range of motion.

Exhausted muscles equal loose ligaments

Research comparing the laxity of the knee among runners, basketball players and weightlifters shows that power lifters who do frequent squats don't put as much pressure on their ligaments as basketball players and runners do, suggesting that it's the constant flexion and extension of the knee – with little chance to relax and recover, especially in distance running – that places greater stress on the joints.[24]

What does running do to cartilage? Some answers may lie in the research done on beagles trained by a special running programme to run more than normal. After some months, the endurance-type running exercise caused a reduction in cartilage, which the researchers believe indicates either a 'disorganization or a reorientation of the ... collagen network'.[25] Although these results may not apply to humans, they do raise obvious concerns. If dogs – which are born to run – can have their cartilage affected by constant running, what does it do to people?

All this evidence raises a couple of fundamentally disturbing questions. Are we, as humans, meant to run for miles on end every day? Are men and women so anatomically different that what's good for one may not be good for the other, particularly without special training?

As always, a middle course may be the most sensible. For men, osteoarthritis is not as much of a worry, but effects on the ligaments may be a possible concern. Just make sure that you include some of the suggestions in the following pages before bursting into a run. To avoid exhausted muscles, think twice before punishing them regularly beyond the minimum for cardiovascular benefit. Consider doing a milder jog.

For women, long punishing daily jogs may be taking your workout too far for knee-joint health and predispose you to arthritis – unless you're prepared to engage in special training to strengthen the muscles supporting the knee.

How runners can prevent knee injury

If you like running or jogging, follow the advice below to minimize the risk of developing arthritis:

Build up your hamstrings: As scientists have discovered, without training, women have significantly different strengths between the hamstring (back thigh) and quadriceps (front thigh) muscles. Before you work out, do regular vertical jumps and ankle jumps (quick bouncing jumps using primarily the lower legs and ankles), and also jump from one leg to the other.

Do exercises that develop strong calf, thigh and ankle muscles, and those around the knee: These all offer vital support for the knee.

Stretch to strengthen your muscles: This is essential before you embark on a running programme. It's vital that you're strong and supple when you start running regularly. For strength training, focus on the hip abductors (the muscles on your outer hips) and external rotator muscles (the six small muscles attached to the top of the thigh bone that allow the hip to rotate sideways).

Develop agility: Exercises to help develop this include making rapid directional changes, which help to develop quick contractions of certain muscles to increase reflex-response time and reduce 'surprise movements' of the joints.

Stay on the flat: Exercise on level surfaces or soft ones like grass.

Replace your running shoes regularly: Change them every three to six months – before they wear out and lose their shock-absorbing capacity.

Pay attention to odd cracking noises in your knees: Most physiotherapists aren't worried by knees that 'click', but if pain, swelling or any other changes develop, these could be the first signs of degenerative joint disease. Get it checked out.

Be versatile: Consider altering your weekly exercise programme so that, besides just running, you introduce other non- or low-impact activities such as swimming, walking or biking.

Building up your knees

To keep the muscles supporting your knees strong and minimize your arthritis risk, both men and women should do the following exercises at least three times a week.

⇨ **Ankle joint flex/extension:** While lying on the floor with your calves propped up on a bench, flex and extend your ankles: 20 times.

⇨ **Calf rises:** Stand with your knees relaxed, hip-width apart. Slowly raise and lower yourself on your toes: 20 times.

⇨ **Lunges:** Take turns with your legs, positioning one leg forward at a 90-degree angle with your front knee bent, keeping your front foot flat on the ground while you position the other leg straight behind: do 5–10 each side.

⇨ **Squat jumps:** Stand with feet shoulder-width apart, arms at sides. Squat (sit back and down like you're about to sit on a chair), moving your arms forward. Keep your knees perpendicular. As you rise, jump up with your arms in the air as though you are reaching for the ceiling. As you land, lower yourself into the squat position again. Do this 10 times. Both squat jumps and lunges will build up your thigh muscles.

Do your knees wobble? Check for knee laxity

If your knees ever feel like they 'give way', get yourself tested with an arthometer. This device measures the 'drawer' movement – the relative position of the lower leg bone to the thighbone. If it can move too far forward – called the 'anterior drawer sign' – you're likely to have loose anterior cruciate ligaments and be more prone to injury to the ligaments and possibly arthritis.

Test the range of motion of all your major joints to determine how loose your ligaments are: a general laxity of joints especially in women has been linked to a tendency for torn ligaments. Test whether you can:

⇨   Touch your thumb to your forearm while your wrist is bent

⇨   Bend forward and place your palms on the floor while keeping your knees straight

⇨   Hyperextend your knee

⇨   Extend your elbow beyond the ordinary range

A 'yes' to any of the above could indicate a greater likelihood to suffer ligament-related injuries.[26] If so, get advice from a trained physiotherapist about proper exercises to compensate. Wear support wraps and choose wisely the level of aerobic activity you want to engage in. But don't stop exercising!

Avoid injuries if possible, and if not ...

Whatever your age, serious injuries to joints – torn ligaments, torn cartilage, or broken bones – can lead to arthritis later in life. For example, people who injure their knees as teenagers and young adults are nearly three times more likely than those without such injuries to have osteoarthritis by the time they reach 65.[27]

Simply being aware of the possibility of injury may be the best way to avoid it. However, if you do sustain an injury during exercise, consider the following alternative treatments:

Take good fats for inflamed joints: The benefits of essential fatty acids (EFAs), particularly omega-3, in the treatment of sore and inflamed joints have been well recognized for many years. While EFAs can't rebuild degenerated cartilage, bone or synovial membranes, they can be effective in relieving the pain and reducing inflammation. Many studies have shown benefits in treating arthritic joints with both omega-3 and omega-6 fatty acids taken as supplements.[28]

Take a glucosamine supplement: Joints require glucosamine, which the body makes from glucose and the amino acid glutamine, to work well and prevent injury. However, those who are very physically active may find it hard to make enough to meet their needs. Most of the research into this supplement has been done with osteoarthritis patients. One study found glucosamine sulphate more effective in relieving pain than the NSAID ibuprofen.[29]

Use the time-honoured RICE method to recover: Rest, Ice, Compression and Elevation.

Walking

Sweat is a great joint lubricant, and one of the best ways to work up a sweat sensibly is by taking a brisk walk. If you haven't exercised a great deal, and depending on the extent of your arthritis, set yourself easy and attainable goals at first. Don't try a mile your first time out. But do walk at least three times a week and steadily increase the pace and length of your outings over time. Wear sensible walking shoes or trainers, and do a few simple stretching exercises to warm up first.

Something to be aware of is the design of your footwear. 'Sensible walking shoes' sounds like a straightforward choice, but not necessarily. In fact, shoes designed to provide additional support are often the very worst things for your knees, and they might even be increasing your chances of developing osteoarthritis. Instead, a new study has discovered that shoes with flexible soles, and even 'flip-flop' sandals, are kinder for your joints.

Researchers at Rush University Medical Center in Chicago made this surprising discovery when they tested four different types of shoes on 31 people with osteoarthritis. They found that special clogs, often worn by healthcare professionals who are on their feet all day, which are designed for comfort, increased the pressure on the wearer's knees compared with flat shoes with flexible soles, and with flip-flops.

The key appears to be the type of sole the shoe has: if it's flexible, it can reduce the load on the knee joints as effectively as medical braces or shoe inserts. Higher heels than basic flat shoes may also be worse for the knee, even when they're part of a special walking shoe.[30]

Cycling

Cycling – either indoors or out – is another great sweat lubricant. Some arthritis sufferers swear that cycling is the answer. Others find it doesn't help their arthritis at all, or even worsens it. It all depends on the individual. Remember, go at your own pace, experiment and see what works for you. If you have arthritis of the hip or knee, a recumbent stationary bike (one on which your legs are not straight under you) may be more comfortable, but still allow rotation and movement.

Swimming

Swimming is the ultimate low-impact exercise. And you don't even have to know how to swim well to enjoy the benefits. Just kicking your legs and sweeping the water with your arms help to loosen and invigorate muscles and joints. And researchers say that this will put enough force on the bones to strengthen them. A Veterans Administration Medical Centre analysis in Portland, Oregon, compared the bones of men who swam to the bones of men who did no exercise, and found that the swimmers had thicker bones. As with walking, set easy goals at first and build up your routine to include a more vigorous workout.

Gardening

Not into going to the gym or heading to the bike trail? How about your own back garden? Researchers find that being in nature is highly relaxing and an anti-stress tonic. Hoeing, weeding and digging are all good bone-building activities. And all the bending and lifting help build flexibility and increase muscle tone. Plus, your garden ends up looking great. Just make sure to use cushions if you have knee arthritis and are kneeling for any length of time.

Take up Tai chi

Tai Chi Chuan is a martial art form that was developed around 1,500 years ago. The version we see practised in parks, a gentle exercise regime that people of all ages can practise, is known as Hand Form, a series of slow movements with the hands that can help keep the mind sharp and the limbs and joints free of aches and pains. Its philosophy is rooted in Traditional Chinese Medicine (TCM), which works with the body's chi, or energy system.

According to doctors of TCM, chi imbalance occurs when the body's energy (chi) is blocked, stagnant, in excess or deficient. Any of these situations can lead to disease, and acupuncture and TCM herbs can help free up blockages and get the chi moving freely again.

Tai chi is a preventative method as its movements keep the chi flowing. It also helps to heal arthritis. And there's plenty of evidence to suggest it really does work – which means it presents a real problem for Western medicine. Its movements are supposed to rebalance yin (feminine/negative electromagnetic charges) and yang (masculine/positive electromagnetic charges) and adjust the body's flow of chi, or qi.

Tai chi is recommended by the UK's National Health Service (NHS), which grudgingly admits it definitely helps arthritis and prevents falls in the elderly. Implausible as it may seem to doctors, there's a stack of evidence proving Tai chi's many benefits. One study concluded that it's a great non-drug way to reduce pain levels, and improve movement and joint stiffness.[31]

Fibromyalgia sufferers have reported feeling less pain and a better quality of life after they practised Tai chi every day for 12 weeks.

Interestingly, the improvements in symptom severity continued for at least three months after they stopped the exercise.[32] Twelve weeks of continued practice seems to be the optimal time for improving arthritis too. One group of 72 women with osteoarthritis said their joint pain and stiffness had improved after three months of daily sessions.[33]

Another osteoarthritis study found that Tai chi relieved joint pain and stiffness, and also promoted positive behaviours such as a healthier diet and better stress management.[34] But perhaps the most impressive effect of Tai chi is its apparent ability to slow bone loss in women with arthritis after the menopause, as documented in a review of six studies.[35]

Yoga also comes highly recommended by some practitioners as a potent way to relieve arthritis symptoms, with specific postures, or asanas, designed to help arthritis, but if you're intending to use it for arthritis relief, make sure to find a qualified practitioner to help you achieve your goals.

Meditation reduces inflammation

Mindfulness meditation can reduce chronic inflammation, which plays a key role in a range of health problems, including heart disease, arthritis and asthma. The technique – which focuses attention on the breath, body sensations and thoughts to keep the attention on the present moment – is one of the most effective ways to reduce the inflammation associated with psychological stress. Researchers from the University of Wisconsin-Madison say it may also be an effective alternative to drugs in people who get no help from pharmaceuticals.

Meditation has been used with other stress-reducing alternatives such as nutrition, physical activity and music therapy. In one experiment, a programme combining the latter three approaches showed that all three reduced psychological and physical stress responses to a similar degree to mindfulness, but that only mindfulness meditation also lowered the inflammation associated with stress.[36]

Clean up your lifestyle

The following simple lifestyle options will also help to ward off joint problems:

Drink pure water

Chlorinated water, which is associated with a higher risk of combined cancers,[37] can cause allergic symptoms from skin rashes to intestinal symptoms, arthritis and headaches. Filtered tap water is better than bottled water in plastic bottles, which can leach plastics from their containers. Well water and spring water are ideal as long as they don't contain a lot of minerals or any bacteria.

Brush your teeth twice a day

Yes, people who don't take good care of their teeth and gums are 70 per cent more likely to develop heart disease than those who brush their teeth twice a day and make regular visits to the dentist. But those with poor oral health are also more likely to suffer high levels of C-reactive protein, a marker of inflammation linked to conditions like arthritis, say researchers from University College London. Doctors are beginning to understand the importance of tooth and gum health, and how it relates to overall health, and a study of 2010 reinforces the point.[38]

There also appears to be some association between periodontal disease and other inflammatory conditions such as rheumatoid arthritis. In a Brazilian study of 39 RA patients and 22 healthy controls, scientists concluded that the typical arthritic patient had fewer teeth, and higher levels of dental plaque and gum disease, than found in the general, non-arthritic population.[39]

Know your chemical sensitivities

Whether it's chemical food additives or gas heating, chemical sensitivities are also linked to arthritis. Consider moving your gas boiler to a covered shelter outdoors and cooking with electricity. Nitrogen dioxide, spewed out by gas cookers and gas- and oil-burning boilers, stays concentrated in the home, particularly in this age of double glazing, and is implicated in arthritis, asthma and other allergies. One American study concluded that gas cookers generate concentrations of nitrogen dioxide of 200–400ppb (parts per billion), which means the average kitchen with a gas cooker has an atmosphere comparable to levels of pollution usually accompanied by government health warnings.

Ditch those implants

Strange as it may seem, silicone gel breast implants and other silicone prostheses may cause arthritis-like symptoms, such as swelling of joints, pain, fever and chronic fatigue. The problem appears to be that they promote antibodies to collagen that have been linked to arthritis.[40] Some, but not all, women have seen arthritic symptoms disappear after having their breast implants removed.

Get connected

Loneliness is an entirely subjective experience. Individuals can have a wide circle of friends and still feel lonely, or have just one or two friends and feel part of a community. Marriage is the single most important relationship most of us have, and the sense of closeness we feel with our partner can determine our sense of isolation or connection.

Two studies make the point of how companionship helps guard against arthritis. The first study of 255 people with rheumatoid arthritis found that those who were happily married felt less pain from their condition. Researchers at Johns Hopkins School of Medicine in Baltimore, Maryland, found that those who had a 'non-distressed' marriage reported lower pain levels than those who were either unmarried or had a 'distressed' marriage.[41]

Attitude is everything

Stress and depression have major impacts on rheumatoid arthritis and juvenile idiopathic arthritis, both of which are chronic inflammatory disorders. Scientists at the Regensburg University Clinic in Germany have demonstrated that stress causes a cascade of biological processes that can make the symptoms of rheumatoid arthritis worse.[42]

This means a smile and a good attitude may well be the easiest protection when it comes to guarding against stress-related inflammation. Sociability, positive emotions and general extroversion have all been associated with greater resistance to inflammatory conditions of many varieties.[43]

Not an extrovert? Not to worry. It seems the trick is to include many of the signs of extroversion into your life, such as thinking positively, keeping connected, and staying energetic and involved in life. And laughter, it appears, really can be the best medicine.

American political journalist and author Norman Cousins suffered from heart disease and severe arthritis (ankylosing spondylitis). Told that he had little chance of surviving, he developed a get-better programme that focused on megadoses of vitamin C and developing a positive attitude. He credits his cure, against all odds, to watching Marx Brothers films for hours on end. 'I made the joyous discovery that 10 minutes of genuine belly laughter had an anesthetic effect and would give me at least two hours of pain-free sleep,' he reported. 'When the pain-killing effect of the laughter wore off, we would switch on the motion picture projector again, and not infrequently it would lead to another pain-free interval.'

Numerous studies show that optimists live longer and are healthier than their pessimistic counterparts. A 2009 study by researchers from the University of Rochester Medical Center in New York discovered that extroverts, particularly those with high engagement in life, had dramatically lower levels of the inflammatory chemical interleukin-6 (IL-6) in their blood.[44] IL-6 is an important indicator of stress, and raised levels have been linked to several inflammatory diseases such as rheumatoid arthritis and coronary heart disease.[45] IL-6 is also highly predictive of mortality, with the risk of death reportedly doubling for people over 65 with the highest levels in their blood compared to those people with the lowest levels (less than 1.9pg/ml) in one study of 1,293 healthy adults over 65.46

According to Benjamin Chapman, the lead researcher in the study, 'Beyond physical activity, some people seem to have this innate energy separate from exercise that makes them intrinsically involved in life.' Perhaps it's this *élan vital* that's playing a health-protecting role.[47]

Chapter 13

AT-A-GLANCE TIPS TO HELP YOU PREVENT OR DEAL WITH ARTHRITIS

Here's a quick-reference checklist summarizing many of the facts and observations outlined in this book. If you've had any history of arthritis, it's recommended that you only follow this programme under the supervision of a qualified, experienced professional. Also, consult a professional with knowledge of nutrition about the doses of supplements to take, since these vary, depending on your individual needs.

For Healthy People Who Want to Avoid Arthritis

⇨ Make sure your neck isn't bent all the time and your computer monitor is at eye level; don't slouch while driving; make sure your posture is supportive of your neck at all times. Consider using a desk that allows you to stand and sit, so that you can vary your positions throughout the day.

⇨ Avoid repetitive motions. If you have to do repetitive work, take frequent breaks, stretch, do neck rolls, wrist and finger exercises, or a little yoga.

⇨ Build up your wrists, elbows and knees with strengthening exercises and weight training to support your joints.

⇨ Regularly do stretching exercises to keep ligaments and muscles flexible.

⇨ Take up a good cardio routine that you enjoy (which means you'll do it) – whether walking, biking, swimming or even dancing. Do a cardio activity at least three times a week.

⇨ Note that for women, long punishing daily jogs may be taking your workout too far for knee-joint health – unless you're prepared to engage in special training to strengthen the muscles supporting the knee.

⇨ If injured, give muscles and joints a chance to heal.

⇨ If you do sustain an injury, use the time-honoured RICE method to recover: Rest, Ice, Compression and Elevation.

⇨ Avoid non-steroidal anti-inflammatory drugs (NSAIDs) such as aspirin and ibuprofen.

⇨ If overweight: lose weight.

⇨ Get on a low-inflammation diet.

Diet guidelines

⇨ Opt for a diet heavy on inflammation-reducing vegetables and fruits.

⇨ Broccoli, leafy greens and brightly coloured vegetables are especially good, as are blueberries, strawberries, red and black raspberries and pineapple.

⇨ Eat yams and sweet potatoes instead of white potatoes.

⇨ Eat deep-water fish (salmon, cod, halibut).

⇨ Eat organic chicken and turkey if you're not vegetarian.

⇨ Eat organic free-range eggs.

⇨ Eliminate processed foods, fried foods, sugar and gluten, artificial sweeteners, MSG, artificial additives, corn, hydrogenated vegetable oils, and all carbonated drinks.

⇨ Eliminate or reduce red meats and dairy, alcohol, cereals, pastas, caffeine.

⇨ Go organic – it's the only way to avoid GMOs (genetically modified organisms) and other synthetic 'foods' that irritate the body and force it into an inflammation mode.

⇨ Cook with extra virgin olive oil (organic) for low-heat cooking; use organic coconut, avocado oil, butter (organic) or ghee for high-heat cooking.

⇨ Balance your omega-6 fatty acids to omega-3 fatty acids in approximately a 4:1 ratio.

Lifestyle guidelines

⇨ Drink pure filtered water (not bottled in plastic) and eliminate fluoride.

⇨ Practise good oral hygiene.

⇨ Get rid of any breast implants.

⇨ Get out and get social – being with people uplifts your mood.

⇨ Keep a positive attitude.

⇨ Take up T'ai chi, yoga and/or mindfulness meditation

If You Have Arthritis

⇨ Sort out your gut. Get tested for candida overgrowth, parasites or a leaky gut, low stomach acid and fructose intolerance, all shown to cause arthritis symptoms.

⇨ Get tested for food and environmental allergies and eliminate allergens from your diet and lifestyle.

⇨ Change your diet to a low-inflammation diet. Avoid the big common allergens like dairy and wheat, red meat, all nightshades, processed foods and foods laden with sugar.

⇨ Drink at least eight glasses of pure water a day.

⇨ Drink fresh ginger juice, extract or tea.

⇨ Take mineral baths with magnesium (Epsom salts).

⇨ Have massage sessions to increase circulation and mitigate the pain of arthritis.

⇨ Consider one or more of the following joint-healthy supplements:

> » Glucosamine: up to 3,200mg/day
>
> » Chondroitin: up to 3,600mg/day
>
> » Bromelaine: 750–1,000mg/day – usually in four divided doses
>
> » Collagen hydrolysate: up to 1,200mg/day
>
> » CH-Alpha
>
> » Hyaluronic acid: 40mg/day
>
> » MSM (methylsulphonylmethane): up to 1,200mg a day in divided dosages
>
> » SAM-e (S-adenosylmethionine): up to 1,200mg/day in divided dosages
>
> » Avocado/soya bean unsaponifiable (ASU)

⇨ Try these nutrition-boosting supplements, which can ease arthritis:

> » Vitamin C: 1–3g/day
>
> » B vitamins: Take a balanced B-complex supplement, and daily doses up to 25mg of B5; 900mg–4g of niacinamide (but under medical supervision and in divided doses throughout the day); and 800mcg each of B12 and folic acid.
>
> » Vitamin D3: 2,000IU/day
>
> » Vitamin B3: 250–500mg/day
>
> » Vitamin E: 1,200 to 1,800IU/day

- » Boron

- » Astaxanthin: 300mg/day

⇨ Try acupuncture, which like all the alternative treatments shows scientific evidence of success

⇨ Try these homeopathic remedies:

- » Benzoic acid for gout-like conditions. Also good for gout: Aconite, Belladonna, Bryonia, Clochicum or Ledum

- » Bryonia Alba for pain with inflammation made worse by movement

- » CalcCarb for arthritic knees

- » Colchicum for arthritis pain made worse by exercise

- » Guaiacum for gout and joint abscesses

- » Hypericum for nerve pain from rheumatoid arthritis

- » Ledum pal for gout and rheumatism

- » Rhus tox when initial painful movement improves with continuous motion

- » Paloondo for rheumatoid arthritis

⇨ Experiment with electromagnetic therapies such as TENS, pulsed electromagnetic fields (PEMFs) or cranial EM stimulation.

⇨ Try energy medicine techniques such as Qigong, Reiki and Therapeutic Touch.

⇨ Look to herbal medicine:

» Bromelain: 750–1,000mg/day – usually in four divided doses

» Black cumin: 1 tsp of black cumin seed oil with meals

» Curcumin: 400–800mg/day

» Ginger: 2–4g of fresh ginger juice, extract or tea daily. Or rub ginger oil directly onto a painful joint

» Meta050: 440mg three times a day for four weeks, followed by 880mg twice a day for a further four weeks

» Pycnogenol®: as directed on product packaging or by a practitioner

» Rosehip powder

» Devil's claw: 750mg three times a day

» Guggul: 500mg/day taken with food

» Traditional Chinese Medicine herbs Shu Guan Wen Jing and Shu Guan Qing Luo

» Cayenne cream

» Willow bark

⇨ If lifestyle and supplements don't end pain and restricted mobility, consider non-surgical surgery, in which doctors use your own stem cells to heal damaged joints.

REFERENCES

Introduction

1. Clin Exp Rheumatol, 1999; 17: S13–9

Part I: The Conventional Approach

Chapter 1: Modern Medicine's Theory of Arthritis

1. Environ Health Perspect, 2010; 118: 957–61
2. Lancet, 1997; 349: 1277–81

Chapter 2: First-line Pain Treatment

1. N Engl J Med, 1991; 325: 87–91
2. Gøtzsche, P. *Deadly Medicines and Organized Crime, How Big Pharma Has Corrupted Healthcare.* Radcliffe Publishing Ltd, 2013
3. Lancet, 1989: 519–22; Osteoarthritis Cartilage, 1999; 7(3): 319–20; Osteoarthritis Cartilage, 1999; 7(3): 343–4; Osteoarthritis Cartilage, 1999; 7(3): 345–7; J Rheumatol, 1995; 22(10): 1941–6; Arthritis Rheum, 2005; 52(10): 3137–42
4. Radcliffe Publishing, 2013
5. Dan Med Bull, 1990; 37: 329–36
6. Clin Evid, 2004; 12: 1702–10
7. Scand J Rheum Suppl, 1992; 92: 21–4
8. Gut, 2002; Suppl 3: III25–30
9. Am J Med, 1998; 105(1B): 31S-38S
10. BMJ, 2011; 342: c7086
11. Gasteroenterology Insights, 2013; 5(1):3

12. Proceedings of the Annual Scientific Meeting of the American College of Gastroenterology, 15 Oct 2007

13. Lancet Neurology, 2007; 6: 487–93

14. Lancet Neurology, 2007; 6: 487–93

15. BMJ, 1995; 310: 827–30

16. BMJ, 2004; 329: 324

17. BMC Medicine, 2006; 4: 22

18. Aliment Pharmacol Ther, 2008; 27: 31–40

19. Lancet, 1996; 348: 1413–6

20. BMJ, 2002; 325: 988

21. Cell Rep, 2014; 8: 1241–7

22. http://www.bccancer.bc.ca/drug-database-site/Drug%20Index/Rituximab_monograph_1Sep2014.pdf

23. N Engl J Med, 1992; 327: 749–54; Gastroenterology, 1993; 104: 1832–47

24. Inflammopharmacology, 2005; 13: 419–25

25. BMJ, 2005; 331: 1310–6

26. Am J Med, 2005; 118: 1271–8

27. JAMA, 2000; 284: 1247–55

28. BMJ, 1999; 319: 1518

29. Tidsskr Nor Laegeforen, 2002; 122: 476–80

30. N Engl J Med, 2005; 352: 1071–80

31. Drug Saf, 2005; 28: 803–16

32. N Engl J Med, 2002; 347: 2104–10

33. Curr Pain Headache Rep, 2005; 9: 377–89

34. www.fda.gov/ForConsumers/ConsumerUpdates/ucm453610.html

Chapter 3: Second-line Treatments

1. Drug Saf, 2002; 25:173–97

2. Arthritis Rheum, 1990; 33: 1449–61

3. N Engl J Med, 1994; 330: 1368–75

4. J Clin Epidemiol, 1993; 46: 315–21

5. Drugs Ther Bull, 1993; 31:18

6. N Engl J Med, 1994; 330: 1368–75

7. Drugs Ther Bull, 1993; 31:18

8. Rheumatology, 2000; 39: 1374–82

9. Ann Rheum Dis, 2001; 60: 566–72

10. Eur J Rheumatol Inflamm, 1991; 11: 148–61

11. Ann Rheum Dis, 1990; 49: 25–7

12. N Engl J Med, 1994; 330: 1368–75; Ann Rheum Dis, 1990; 49: 25-7

13. Drugs Ther Bull, 1993; 31:18

14. Cannon GW, Ward JR. 'Cytotoxic drugs and sulfasalazine', in McCarty DJ, ed. *Arthritis and Allied Conditions*. Philadelphia, PA: Lea & Febiger, 1989

15. Ann Rheum Dis, 1985; 44: 194–8

16. Ann Rheum Dis, 1985; 44: 194–8

17. J Rheumatol Suppl, 1988; 16: 9–13

18. Drugs Ther Bull, 1993; 31:18

19. Arthritis Rheum, 1979; 22: 832

20. APLAR J Rheumatol, 2006; 9: 165–9

21. Medicine (Baltimore), 2005; 84: 291–302; Prescrire Int, 2004; 13: 171–5

22. Expert Opin Drug Saf, 2005; 4: 637–41

23. Arthritis Rheum, 2005; 52: 2513–8

24. Prescrire Int, 2004; 13: 171–5

25. Rheumatology (Oxford), 2005; 44: 714–20

26. Rev Mal Respir, 2004; 21: 1107–15

27. Neth J Med, 2005; 63: 112–4

28. Expert Opin Drug Saf, 2005; 4: 637–41

29. Ann Intern Med, 2008; 148(2): 124–34

30. J Pharmacol Pharmacother, 2013; 4 (Suppl 1): S94–8

31. Br J Ophthalmol, 1998; 82: 704–8

32. Ann Intern Med, 1993; 15; 963–8

33. Allergy Asthma Clin Immunol, 2011; 7: 13

34. Arthroscopy, 1985; 1: 68–72

35. JAMA Intern Med. 2013; 173(6):444-9

Chapter 4: Operations for Arthritis

1. Arthritis Rheum, 1993; 36: 289–96

2. N Engl J Med, 2002; 347: 81–8

3. J Bone Joint Surg Am, 2001; 83-A: 1524–8; Acta Orthop Scand, 2000; 71: 19–27

4. Arch Intern Med, 2002; 162: 1465–71

5. J Bone Joint Surg Br, 1994; 76-B: 701–12

6. N Engl J Med, 1996; 335: 133–4

7. Curr Opin Rheumatol, 1994; 6: 172–6

8. J Bone Joint Surg Br, 1988; 70: 539–42

9. J Natl Cancer Inst, 2001; 93: 1405–10

10. J Bone Joint Surg Am, 1997; 79: 1599–617

11. J Bone Joint Surg Br, 1995; 77-B: 520–7

12. Lancet, 2012; 379: 1199–1204

13. Clin Orthop, 1996; 329 Suppl: S78-88; Clin Orthop, 2000; 379: 123-33

14. Acta Orthop, 2007; 78(6) :746–54; J Arthroplasty, 2006; 21(6 suppl 2):17–25

15. J Bone Joint Surg Br, 1999; 81(5): 835–42; Acta Orthop Scand, 1998; 69: 253–8; Clin Orthop, 2001; 393: 112–20

16. JAMA, 1994; 271: 1349–57

17. J Bone Joint Surg Am, 1991; 73(6): 848–57

18. Arthritis Rheumatol, 2014; 66: 2134–43

19. Instr Course Lect, 2008; 57: 383–413

20. Foot Ankle Int, 2000; 21: 182–94

21. J Am Acad Orthop Surg, 2000; 8: 200–9

22. J Bone Joint Surg Am, 2003; 85: 923–36

23. J Bone Joint Surg Am, 2007; 89(9):1899-905

24. J Bone Joint Surg Am, 2001; 83-A: 219–28

25. J Bone Joint Surg Am, 2006; 88: 526–35; Acta Orthop Scand, 1981; 52: 103–5

26. J Bone Joint Surg Br, 2005; 87-B: 343–7

27. Foot Ankle Int, 2008; 29: 3–9; Acta Orthop Scand, 1981; 52: 103–5

28. American Orthopaedic Society for Sports Medicine, news release, 15 Mar 2014

29. N Engl J Med, 2002; 347: 81–8

Part II: The Dietary Approach to Arthritis

Chapter 5: It's Not Old Age, It's Inflammation

1. http://med.stanford.edu/ism/2011/november/osteoarthritis.html

2. Nat Med, 2011; 17: 1674–9

3. Ann Allergy, 1949; 7: 200

4. Lancet, 1986; 1: 236–8

5. Lancet, 1991; 338: 899–902

6. J Neurol Orthop Med Surg, 1993; 12: 227–31

7. J Neurol Orthop Med Surg, 1993; 12: 227–31; J Intern Acad Prev Med, 1979; 7: 31–7

8. Arthritis Res Ther, 2006; 8 (Suppl 1): S2; Br J Rheumatol, 1987; 26: 303–6

9. Toxicology, 1992; 73: 127–46

10. Crit Rev Eukaryot Gene Expr, 2011; 21: 131–42; Basic Clin Pharmacol Toxicol, 2014; 114: 103–8

11. Arthritis Rheum, 2012; 64: 2927–36

12. Nutr Metab (Lond), 2010; 7: 32

13. www.sciencedaily.com/releases/2010/01/100125123231.htm

14. J Autoimmun, 1994; 7: 775–89

15. Clin Exp Rheumatol, 1990; 8: 75–83

16. Gut, 1986; 27: 1292–1297

17. Gut, 1998; 43(4): 506–11

18. Elife, 2013; 2: e01202

19. Basic Health Publications, 2nd edition, 2014; or see their website at: www.groundology.com/research/thermographic_histories_2004.pdf

Chapter 6: The Secret Connection: Your Gut

1. J Adv Med, 1993; 6: 67–82; Clin Dev Immunol, 2013; 2013: 872632; Autoimmune Dis, 2012; 2012: 539282; Clin Diagn Lab Immunol, 1997; 4(4): 393–9

2. Baillieres Clin Rheumatol, 1989; 3: 271–84

3. Gut, 1986; 27: 1292–7

4. Br J Rheumatol, 1992; 31: 443–7

5. Nature, 2012; 487: 104–8

6. J Am Diet Assoc, 2006; 106: 1631–9

7. J Clin Gastroenterol, 2008; 42: 233–8; J Pediatr Gastroenterol Nutr, 2008; 47: 303–8

8. J Am Diet Assoc, 2009; 109: 1204–14; Curr Gastroenterol Rep, 2009; 11: 368–74

9. Allergy, 1991; 66: 181–4

10. Surgery, 1990; 107: 411–6; Allergy, 1989; 44 Suppl 9: 47–51; Ann Allergy, 1991; 66: 181–4

11. Lancet, 1984; 1: 179–82; Gut, 1991; 32: 66–9; Eur J Pediatr, 1988; 147: 123–7

12. Toxicol Appl Pharmacol, 1992; 114(2): 285–94; Food Chem Toxicol, 1999; 37(6):627–37; Food Chem Toxicol, 2014; 74: 349–59; Cell Biol Toxicol, 2005; 21(3–4): 163–79

13. Lancet, 1993; 341: 843–8

14. J Nutr, 1983; 113: 2300–7

15. PLoS ONE, 2007; 2(12): e1308; Am J Pathol, 2012; 180(2): 626–35

16. Arch Surg, 1990; 125: 1040–5

17. Am J Clin Nutr, 1991; 54: 346–50

18. Am J Gastroenterol, 1989; 84: 1285–7; Gastroenterology, 1989; 96: 981–8

19. Torgan, C. 'Gut Microbes Linked to Rheumatoid Arthritis', NIH Research Matters, 25 Nov 2013

20. Evid Based Complement Alternat Med, 2014; 2014: 159819; Tokai J Exp Clin Med, 1990; 15: 417–23; J Infect Dis, 1987; 155: 979–84; Nature, 1967; 215: 527–8

21. Acta Gastroenterol Latinoam, 1988; 18: 195–201

22. Clin Microbiol Rev, 2006; 19: 50–62; Phytomedicine, 2009; 16: 972–5; J Appl Bacteriol, 1989; 66: 69–75

23. Gut, 1992; 33: 987–93; Med Microbiol Immunol, 1977; 163: 53–60; Am J Clin Nutr, 1978; 32: 1592–6; Acta Trop, 1979; 36: 147–50

24. Int Immunol, 2004; 16(12): 1761–8

25. Alcohol Clin Exp Res, 1993; 17: 552–5

26. Phytother Res, 2010; 24: 1423–32; J Hepatol, 1989; 9: 105–13

Chapter 7: The Role of Diet

1. Ann Rheumatic Dis, 2003; 62: 208–14

2. Rheumatol, 2001; 40: 1175–9

3. BMJ Open, 2013 (19 Jul); 3(7): pii: e002993

4. Ann Rheum Dis, 2000; 59: 631–5

5. Fluoride, 1998; 31: 13–20

6. Arthritis Rheum, 2013; 65: 3130–40

7. Theor Appl Genet, 2003; 106(4): 727–34

8. Proc Nutr Soc. 2014; 73(2): 278–88; Int J Mol Sci, 2013; 14(11): 23063–85

9. Arthritis Res Ther, 2006; 8 (Suppl 1): S2; Epub 2006 Apr 12; Adv Exp Med Biol, 1974; 41: 443–449; J Chronic Dis, 1976; 29: 793–800

10. Arthritis Rheum, 2012; 64(12): 4004–11; J Nutr, 2003; 133: 1826–9

11. Lancet, 1991; 338: 899–902; Scand J Rheumatol, 1995; 24: 85–93

12. Clin Rheumatol, 1994; 13: 475–82

13. Scand J Rheumatol, 2001; 30(1): 1–10

14. Am J Clin Nutr. 1999; 70(3 Suppl): 594S–600S

15. Cell Stem Cell, 2014; 14: 810–23

16. Laver, M. *Diet for Life.* Pan, 1981

Chapter 8: Healing with Essential Fatty Acids

1. Circulation, 2009; 119: 902–907

2. Circulation, 1999; 99: 779–85

3. Circulation, 2006; 113: 2062–70

4. N Engl J Med, 2004; 350: 29–37

5. Am J Clin Nutr, 1996; 63: 698–703

6. Cancer Epidemiol Biomarkers Prev, 2008; 17: 2748–54

7. Circulation, 2000; 102; 2677–9; Pharmacol Res, 1999; 40: 211–25; Cardiovasc Res, 2001; 52: 361–371; Circulation, 2002; 106: 2747–57

8. Am J Clin Nutr, 1991; 54: 438–63; Am J Clin Nutr, 2000; 71: 171S–5S

9. Am J Clin Nutr, 1991; 54: 438–63

10. Prog Lipid Res, 2003; 42: 544–56

11. Am J Clin Nutr, 1991; 54: 438–63

12. Lancet, 1994; 343: 1268–71

13. J Clin Epidemiol, 1995; 48(11): 1379–90

14. Arch Med Res, 2012; 43(5): 356–62

15. Epidemiol, 1996; 7(3): 256–63

16. J Am Coll Nutr, 2007; 26: 39–48

17. Am J Clin Nutri, 1999; 70: 1077–1082

18. J Rheumatol, 2002; 29: 1708–12

19. J Rheumatol, 2004; 31: 767–74

20. J Strength Cond Res, 2005; 19: 115–21

21. J Strength Cond Res, 2005; 19: 475–80

22. Inflammopharmacology, 1997; 5: 127–32

Part III: Alternative Treatments for Arthritis

Chapter 9: The Best Alternatives

1. J of Clin Nurs, 2012; 21: 3198–204

2. Acta Anaesthesiolog Scand, 1992; 36(6): 519–25

3. Acupunct Med, 2001; 19(1): 19–26

4. Life Sci, 2002; 71(2): 191–204

5. Evid Based Complement Alternat Med, 2005; 2: 79–84

6. Am J Chin Med, 2001; 29: 187–99

7. J Altern Complement Med, 2009; 15: 613–8; MMW Fortschr Med, 2007; 149: 37–9

8. Acupunct Med, 2012; Doi:10.1136/acupmed-2012-010151

9. Arch Intern Med, 2012; 10: 1–10

10. J Tradit Chin Med, 2004; 24: 185–7

11. Br Homeopath J, 1986; 75: 148-57

12. The Center for Integrative Medicine, The Encyclopedia of New Medicine, London: Rodale Books, 2006

13. Rheum Dis Clin North Am, 2000; 26(1): 51–62

14. Altern Ther Health Med, 2001; 7(5): 54–64, 66–9

15. Cochrane Database Syst Rev, 2013; 12: CD003523

16. J Rehabil Res Dev, 2007; 44: 195–222

17. Pain, 2007; 130: 157–65; Curr Opin Anaesthesiol, 2009; 22(5): 623–6

18. Biomed Pharmacother, 2005; 59(7): 388–94

19. J Clin Rheumatol, 2001; 7: 72–8; J Rehabil Res Dev, 2006; 43: 461–74

20. J Rehabil Res Dev, 2007; 44: 195–222

21. Altern Ther Health Med, 1999; 5(1): 45–54

22. J Pain, 2007; 8: 827–31

23. Evid Based Complement Alternat Med, 2004; 1(3): 251–7

24. Clin Exp Rheumatol, 2006; 24: 25–30

25. Altern Med Rev, 2010; 15: 361–8

26. Altern Med Rev, 2010; 15: 361–8

27. Int Immunopharmacol, 2005; 5: 1749–70

28. Phytother Res, 2012; 26(8): 1246–8

29. Inflamm Res, 2009; 58: 899–908; Altern Med Rev, 2010; 15: 337–44

30. J Med Food, 2005; 8: 125–32

31. Phytother Res, 2005; 19: 864–9

32. Phytother Res, 2008; 22: 1087–92

33. Scand J Rheumatol, 2005; 34: 302–8

34. Rheumatology, 2001; 40: 779–93; MMW Fortschr Med, 2007; 149: 51–6

35. J Ethnopharmacol, 1991; 33: 91–5

36. Minerva Gastroenterol Dietol, 2015 (22 Oct); Epub ahead of print PubMed PMID: 26492586

37. BMC Complement Alt Med, 2004; 4: 13

38. Altern Ther Health Med, 2003; 9(3): 74–9

39. J Tradit Chin Med, 2000; 20(2): 87–92
40. Semin Arthritis Rheum, 2005; 34: 773–84
41. J Inflamm (Lond), 2006; 3: 6
42. J Inflamm (Lond), 2006; 3: 6
43. Arzneimittelforschung, 2001; 51: 896–903
44. J Rheumatol, 1992; 19: 604–7
45. Cochrane Database Syst Rev, 2006; 2: CD004504

Chapter 10: Super Supplements for Arthritis

1. Altern Med Rev, 2004; 9: 275–96
2. Ann Rheum Dis, 2011; 70: 982–9
3. Osteoarthritis Cartilage, 2008; 16 Suppl 3: S19–21
4. Med Hypotheses, 2000; 54(5): 798–802
5. Lancet, 2001; 357: 251–56
6. Lancet, 2001; 357: 247
7. Clin Ther, 1980; 3: 260–72
8. Ann Rheum Dis, 2016; 75: 37–44
9. Sci Rep, 2015; 5: 16827
10. Arthritis Rheumatol, 2015; 67 (S10): 1–4046 (abstr 950)
11. J Res Pharm Pract, 2013; 2: 34–9
12. Curr Med Res Opin, 2006; 22: 2221–32; Complement Ther Med, 2012; 20(3): 124–30
13. Osteoarthritis Cartilage, 2007; 15: C61–2
14. *See* www.betterjoints.com/clinical-evidence
15. Orthopäd Prax, 2005; 41: 486–94
16. Drugs R D, 2011; 11: 13–27
17. World J Gastroenterol, 2007; 13: 945–9
18. Nutr J, 2008; 7: 3
19. Cochrane Database Syst Rev, 2006; 2: CD005321; Osteoarthritis Cartilage, 2006; 14: 867–74
20. BMC Complement Altern Med, 2011; 11: 50
21. Clin Ther, 2009; 31: 2860–72
22. Am J Med, 1987; 83: 81–3; Am J Med, 1987; 83: 66–71
23. Crit Rev Food Sci Nutr, 2008; 48: 458–63
24. Osteoarthritis Cartilage, 2008; 16: 399–408; Rheumatology, 2001; 40: 779–93; Clin Rheumatol, 1998; 17: 31–9

25. Br J Nutr, 2001; 85(3): 251–69; Analyst, 1998; 123(1): 3–6

26. Br J Nutr, 2001; 85: 251–69

27. J Rheumatol, 1997; 24(4): 643–6

28. Arthritis Rheum, 1996; 39: 648–56

29. J Am Geriatr Soc, 1978; 26: 328–30; Ther Adv Musculoskelet Dis, 2012; 4: 11–19

30. Arthritis Rheum, 1991; 34: 1205–6; Ann Rheum Dis, 1997; 56: 649–55

31. J Am Geriatr Soc, 1955; 3: 927–36; Inflam Res, 1996; 45: 330–4

32. J Am Coll Nutr, 1994; 13: 351–6

33. Arthritis Rheum, 1990; 33: 9–18

34. J Nutr Med, 1990; 1: 127–32

35. Crit Rev Food Sci Nutr, 2003; 43: 219–31

36. Am J Physiol, 1992; 263: R734–7

37. Ann Rheum Dis, 2009; 68: 817–22

38. Pain Med, 2008; 9: 979–84

39. www.vitamind3world.com/vitamin_D_for_chronic_pain.pdf

40. Spine, 2003; 28: 177–9

41. J Rehabil Res Dev, 2007; 44: 195–222; Wien Med Wochenschr, 1999; 149: 577–80

42. Prog Clin Biol Res, 1985; 192: 363–70

43. BMC Complement Altern Med, 2004; 4: 13

Chapter 11: Non-Surgical Surgery

1. J Bone Joint Surg Am, 2010; 92: 994–1009; Arthritis Res Ther, 2009; 11: 211

2. Eur Cell Mater, 2005; 9: 23–32

3. J Bone Joint Surg Br, 2001; 83: 289–94

4. Arthritis Rheum, 2007; 56: 1175–86; Best Pract Res Clin Rheumatol, 2008; 22: 269–84

5. Pain Physician, 2008; 11: 343–53

6. Curr Stem Cell Res Ther, 2011; 6(4): 368–78

Chapter 12: Lifestyle for Healthy Joints

1. Purves D et al., eds. *Neuroscience*, 2nd edn Sunderland, MA: Sinauer Associates, 2001

2. Rev Med Suisse, 2009; 5: 1380–2, 1384–5

3. Int J Clin Exp Hypn, 2000; 48: 138–53

4. Behav Med, 2006; 29(1): 95–124

5. Rev Med Suisse, 2009; 5: 1380–2, 1384–5

6. Int J Clin Hypn, 2006; 54(4):432–47

7. Pract Pain Manage, 2003; 3: 12–18; Pain Med, 2014 Apr; 15 Suppl 1:S21–39

8. Cochrane Database Syst Rev, 2004; 1: CD000447

9. Cochrane Database Syst Rev, 2012; 9: CD008880. Cochrane Database Syst Rev, 2011; 2: CD008112.

10. Cochrane Database Syst Rev, 2008; 4: CD001929

11. J Altern Complement Med, 2003; 9: 837–46

12. J Rehabil Res Dev, 2007; 44: 195–222

13. Agents Actions, 1976; 6(4): 454–9

14. Ann Rheum Dis, 1975; 34(4): 340–5

15. Ann Agric Environ Med, 2013; 20(2): 312–6

16. K D Rainsford, in J R J Sorensen, ed., Inflammatory Diseases and Copper, New York, NY: Humana Press, 1982

17. Weleda, product code 6066

18. Diabetologia, 2010; 53(6): 1217–26

19. Analyst, 1998; 123(1): 3–6

20. Eur J Phys Rehabil Med, 2016 (19 Feb) (Epub ahead of print) PubMed PMID: 26899038; Int J Biometeorol, 2016 (26 Jan) (Epub ahead of print) PubMed PMID: 26813884; J Rheumatol, 1994; 21: 1305–9; Rheumatol Int, 2001; 20(3): 105–8

21. JAMA, 1997; 277: 25–31; Arch Intern Med, 2005; 165: 2355–60; Am Fam Physician, 2002; 65: 419–26

22. Arthritis Rheum, 1996; 39: 988–95

23. J Electromyogr Kinesiol, 2004; 14: 475–83

24. Am J Sports Med, 1986; 14: 24–9

25. Ann Rheum Dis, 1996; 55: 253–64

26. Orthopaedics, 2005; 28: 656–60

27. Ann Intern Med, 2000; 133: 321–8

28. Eur J Clin Invest, 1992; 22: 687–91; Arthritis Rheum, 1995; 38: 1107–14; Br J Rheumatol, 1994; 33: 847–52; Arthritis Rheum, 1996; 39: 1808–17

29. Curr Med Res Opin, 1982; 8: 145–9

30. Arthritis Care Res, 2010; Doi: 10.1002/acr.20165

31. BMJ Open, 2011; 1: e000035

32. N Engl J Med, 2010; 363: 743–54

33. J Rheumatol, 2003; 30: 2039–44

34. Taehan Kanho Hakhoe Chi, 2007; 37: 249–56

35. Arch Phys Med Rehabil, 2007; 88: 673–80

36. Brain Behav Immun, 2013; 27: 174–84

37. Am J Publ Health, 1992; 82: 955–63

38. BMJ, 2010; 340: c2451

39. Braz Oral Res, 2008; 22: 72–7

40. J Autoimmune, 1993; 6: 367–77; J Autoimmune, 1994; 7: 775–89

41. J Pain, 2010; 11: 958–64

42. Med Klin (Munich), 2005; 100: 794–803

43. Psychol Sci, 2003; 14: 389–95; Psychosom Med, 2003; 65: 652–7; Health Psychol, 2001; 20: 4–11; Neurology, 2009; 72: 253–9

44. Brain Behav Immun, 2009; 23: 636–42

45. Ann Intern Med, 1998; 128: 127–37; Atherosclerosis, 2000; 148: 209–14

46. Am J Med, 1999; 106: 506–12

47. Brain Behav Immun, 2009; 23: 636–42

ACKNOWLEDGEMENTS

E very book is a collective activity, and none more so than this one, which bears the silent fingerprints of a raft of people involved with What Doctors Don't Tell You, the publication and website, since its beginnings in 1989.

Much of the information contained in this book represents the best material gathered over the years about arthritis by a number of WDDTY writers and editors, and published in one form or another in our newsletter magazine, or on our website. They include, chiefly, Bryan Hubbard, Lynne McTaggart and Joanna Evans, but also Dr Harald Gaier, WDDTY's Medical Detective. We are also indebted to a number of doctors and practitioners for their help with research and ideas, particularly Dr John Mansfield.

Thanks are particularly due to Cate Montana, who was involved in the initial assembly of this material; Emilie Crosier, for crosschecking the facts and hundreds of references cited in this book; and Jo Evans, for some last-minute edits and additions.

The entire Hay House team has our deep gratitude for their enthusiastic and courageous embracing of this project, but most particularly Reid Tracy, Michelle Pilley, Julie Oughton and Jo

Burgess. We are also indebted to Bob Saxton and Lucy Buckroyd, for their careful copyediting and suggestions, which improved the manuscript in countless ways.

Finally we are grateful to the other members of WDDTY's indefatigable UK team, who add to its mission in countless ways, including Jimmy Egerton, Sharyn Wong, Trevor Jayakody, Laura Ramsay, Kelly-Marie During, Buster Manston, Mark Jones, Bruce Sawford, Emilie Crosier, Rick Greer and our teams at Comag and Esco who handle distribution and subscriptions.

Two others are responsible, in a sense, for the birth of this manuscript. As a young journalist, one of us (Lynne) was privileged to edit the work of Dr Robert Mendelsohn, whose prescient views about medicine initially influenced both of us. We were also extremely fortunate to have come across Dr Stephen Davies, the nutritional pioneer who not only successfully treated Lynne's condition but also helped us to view disease and the means to treat it in a completely new light. They were the midwives who gave birth to what has become a major focus of our journalistic work – what we have come to believe is the biggest, most important story of all.

INDEX

NOTES